T0257130

Piet de Boer
Steven J Morgan
Christian van der Werken

Handbook

Orthopaedic
Trauma Care

Piet de Boer
Steven J Morgan
Christian van der Werken

Handbook

Orthopaedic
Trauma Care

650 illustrations

 Thieme

Library of Congress Cataloging-in-Publication Data is available from the publisher.

The content of this book is based on a translation of the book "Letsels van het steun- en
bewegingsapparaat", copyright © 2000 Reed Business Information bv, Maarssen, The Netherlands
Copyright © 2009 English translation: AO Publishing, Switzerland, Clavadelerstrasse 8,
CH-7270 Davos Platz
Distribution by Georg Thieme Verlag, Rüdigerstrasse 14, DE-70469 Stuttgart and Thieme New York,
333 Seventh Avenue, US-New York, NY 10001

ISBN 9783131468710
E-ISBN 9783131470317

Table of contents

Introduction

The Handbook of Orthopaedic Trauma Care is intended for physicians and other healthcare professionals in charge of the immediate management of patients suffering from trauma. This book is designed to provide them with the vital information needed for the immediate assessment and management of these patients in a concise and easily understandable structure.

This handbook gives basic information as to how bone and soft-tissue injuries heal and how medical care can influence this process. Specific injuries are discussed region by region throughout the body and the pathologies described not only cover fractures and dislocations but also soft-tissue injuries. Each chapter in turn is divided into individual pathologies and information is given as to the mechanism of the injury, clinical presentation, diagnostics, classification, treatment, duration of injury, and prognosis. The text is complimented by simple illustrations showing key clinical points in the management of trauma patients.

The Handbook of Orthopaedic Trauma Care was developed from an earlier book in Dutch titled "Letsels van het steun- en bewegingsapparaat" by Prof Dr Christian van der Werken (ed), Prof Peter RG Brink, Prof Dr Henk J Klasen, Dr Sam de Lange, Prof Dr René K Marti, Dr Ad JG Nollen, Dr Ernst LFB Raaijmakers, and Dr Luuk S de Vries that was published in 2000 by Elsevier. Later the rights of translation of that book were granted by Elsevier to AO Publishing. The content and illustrations have been updated and reworked by an international group of trauma surgeons to reflect changes in practice.

We hope that this book will provide invaluable support to physicians and other healthcare professionals when faced with emergency situations about which they may not be familiar. We believe that the information presented will allow the healthcare professional to make more rapid and accurate decisions, which in turn will result in a higher standard of care.

Piet de Boer, MA, FRCS
Steven J Morgan, MD, FACS
Christian van der Werken, Prof, MD, PhD
2009

Editors and contributors

Piet de Boer, MA FRCS
Education
AO Foundation
Dübendorf, Switzerland

Doug A Campbell, ChM, FRCS Ed, FRCS(Orth), FFSEM (UK)
Consultant Hand and Wrist Surgeon
Leeds Teaching Hospitals NHS Trust
Leeds, United Kingdom

Klaus Dresing, Prof Dr med
Assistant Medical Director
University Medicine Göttingen Georg-August-Universität
Göttingen, Germany

Michael Erler, MD
Chafers Hospital for Trauma and Reconstructive Surgery
St Georg Eisenach GmbH
Eisenach, Germany

Christopher G Finkemeier, MD, MBA
Co-Director Orthopaedic Trauma Surgeons of California
Roseville, CA, USA

David F Hubbard, MD, Prof
Department of Orthopaedic Surgery
Chief, Section of Orthopaedic Trauma
West Virginia University School of Medicine
Morgantown, WV, USA

Mauricio Kfuri Jr, MD
Depto Biomecânica, Medicina e Reabilitação do Ap. Locomotor
Faculdade de Medicina de Ribeirão Preto - USP
Ribeirão Preto-SP, Brazil

Kodi E Kojima, MD, PhD
Chief of Orthopaedic Trauma Group
Santa Casa Medical School
Sao Paulo, Brazil

Tak Wing Lau, MD
Department of Orthopaedics and Traumatology
Queen Mary Hospital,
Pokfulam,
Hong Kong

Cong-Feng Luo MD, PhD
Professor and Chief
Department of Orthopaedic Trauma III
Shanghai Sixth People's Hospital
Shanghai JiaoTong University
Shanghai, P.R. China

Steven Morgan, MD, FACS
Associate Director of Orthopaedics
Denver Health Medical Center
Associate Professor & Orthopaedic Residency Program Director
University of Colorado School of Medicine
Denver, CO, USA

Ananda M Nanu
M S(Orth) M Ch Orth FRCS FRCS Orth
Consultant Trauma and Orthopaedic Surgeon
Sunderland Royal Hospitals
Sunderland, United Kingdom

Jong-Keon Oh, MD
Department of Orthopaedic Surgery
Korea University Guro Hospital
Seoul, Korea

F Cumhur Öner, MD, PhD
University Medical Center
Department of Orthopaedic Surgery
Utrecht, The Netherlands

Martin D Richardson, MBBS, MS, FRACS
University of Melbourne
Department of Surgery
Royal Melbourne Hospital
Victoria, Australia

Wa'el S Taha, ABO
Assistant Professor of Surgery
Consultant Orthopaedic Trauma
King Abdulaziz Medical City
Riyadh, Saudi Arabia

Christian van der Werken, Prof, MD, PhD
University Medical Center
Department of Surgery
Utrecht, The Netherlands

1 Principles

1 Principles

1.1 Fracture classification

"A classification is useful only if it considers the severity of the bone lesion and serves as a basis for treatment and for evaluation of the results" (Maurice E Müller, 1988).

Goals of fracture classification systems:
- Evaluate the injury systematically
- Assist surgeons in developing a treatment plan for specific fractures
- Predict the expected outcome
- Facilitate communication among physicians
- Assist in documentation and research

Of many classification systems that have been proposed so far, the Müller AO Classification of fractures–long bones is one that is most widely accepted and used.

1.2 Müller AO Classification of Fractures–Long Bones

The Müller AO Classification of Fractures–Long Bones use a five-element alphanumeric code.

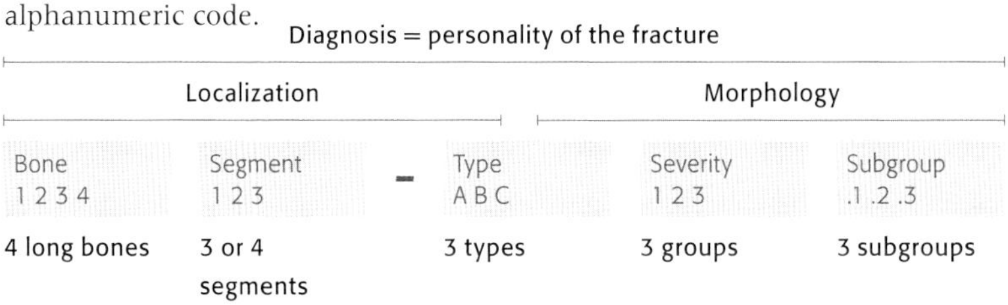

Diagnosis = personality of the fracture

Localization			Morphology	
Bone 1 2 3 4	Segment 1 2 3	— Type A B C	Severity 1 2 3	Subgroup .1 .2 .3
4 long bones	3 or 4 segments	3 types	3 groups	3 subgroups

Fig 1-1   Alphanumeric structure of the Müller AO Classification of fractures–long bones.

To make full use of this system, we need to recognize, identify, and describe the injury to the bone according to the defined terminology. This description can then be converted to an alphanumeric code for documentation and research purposes.

1.3   Description of fractures

To accurately describe a fracture we need to define its location and characteristics or morphology.

Location

The location can be described with the bone and segment concept. The anatomical location is designated by two numbers: one for the bone and one for its segment.

Bone: 1 Humerus   2 Radius/ulna   3 Femur   4 Tibia/fibula
Segment: 1 Proximal   2 Diaphyseal   3 Distal   4 Malleolar

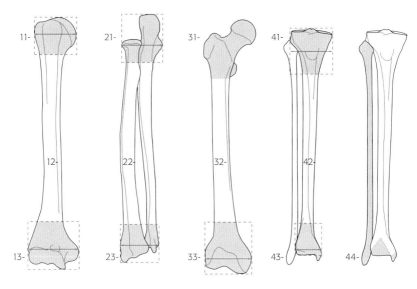

Fig 1-2 Anatomical location of the fracture is designated by two numbers: one for the bone and one for its segment (ulna and radius as well as tibia and fibula are regarded as one bone). The patella and the malleolar segments are assigned segment 4 as 34 and 44, respectively. Proximal or distal segments are defined by a square which has the same length as the widest part of the epiphysis (exceptions 31 and 44).

Determination of the center of the fracture

Before a fracture can be assigned to a segment the center must first be determined. In a simple fracture, the center of the fracture is going to be the center of a spiral or oblique fracture line. In a wedge fracture, the center is the broadest part of the wedge. In a complex fracture, the center can only be determined after reduction.

If the fracture is associated only with an undisplaced fissure which reaches the joint, it is classified as metaphyseal or diaphyseal depending on where its center is.

By assigning numbers for each bone and segments, the location of the fracture can then be expressed with two numbers.

Morphology: type, group, subgroup

  ■ The morphology of the fracture is described according to a defined terminology.

All fractures are either simple or multifragmentary.

Simple: A term used to characterize a single circumferential disruption of a diaphysis or metaphysis, or a single disruption of an articular surface. Simple fractures of the diaphysis or metaphysis are spiral, oblique, or transverse.

Multifragmentary: A term used to characterize any fracture with one or more completely separated intermediate fragments. In the diaphyseal and metaphyseal segments, it includes the wedge and the complex fractures.

Wedge: A fracture with one or more intermediate fragments in which, after reduction, there is some contact between the main fragments.

Complex: A fracture with one or more intermediate fragments in which, after reduction, there is no contact between the main proximal and distal fragments.

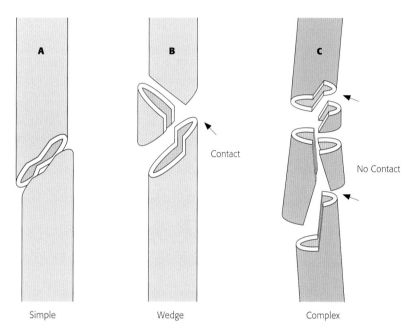

Contact

No Contact

Simple　　　　　　　Wedge　　　　　　　Complex

Fig 1-3　A simple fracture has one fracture line and cortical contact exceeds 90% after reduction. A wedge fracture has three or more fragments, and main fragments have contact after reduction. Complex fractures have no contact between main fragments after reduction.

Description of fractures involving diaphyseal segment

Type: simple (A)
          wedge (B)
          complex (C)

Group: simple (A)   → spiral (A1), oblique (A2), transverse (A3)
          wedge (B)   → spiral wedge (B1), bending wedge (B2),
                           fragmented wedge (B3)
          complex (C)   → spiral (C1), segmental (C2), irregular (C3)

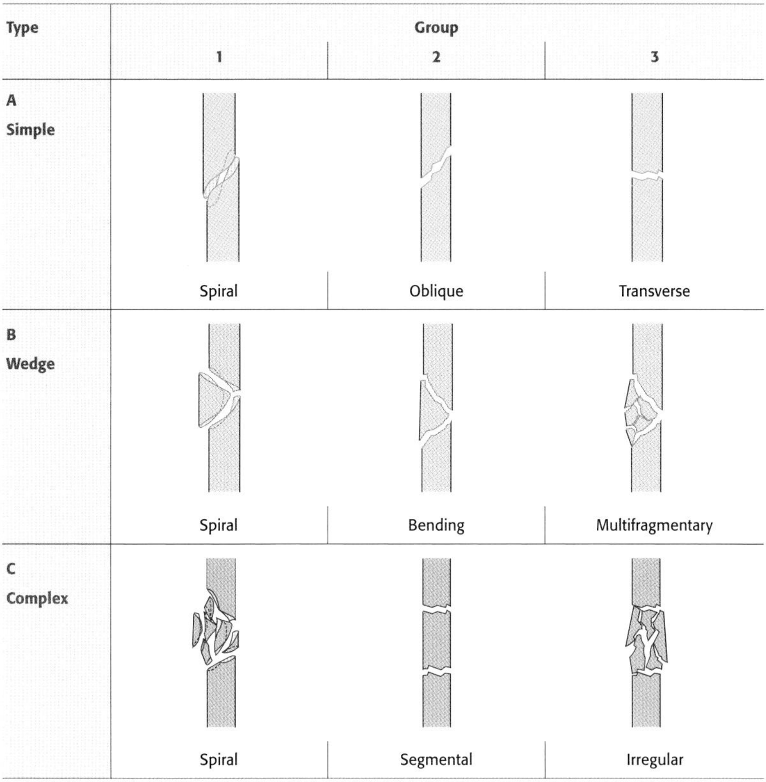

Type	Group		
	1	**2**	**3**
A **Simple**	Spiral	Oblique	Transverse
B **Wedge**	Spiral	Bending	Multifragmentary
C **Complex**	Spiral	Segmental	Irregular

Fig 1-4   Description of diaphyseal fractures.

Specific terms for end segments

Extraarticular fractures (A): Do not involve the articular surface, although they may be intracapsular.

Articular fractures: They are subdivided into partial and complete.

Partial articular fractures (B): Involve only part of the articular surface, while the rest of that surface remains attached to the diaphysis.

Complete articular fractures (C): The articular surface is disrupted and completely separated from the diaphysis. The severity of these fractures depends on whether their articular and metaphyseal components are simple or multifragmentary.

- **C1:** complete articular fracture in which both metaphyseal and articular components are simple.
- **C2:** complete articular fracture in which the metaphyseal component is multifragmentary (complex) and the articular component is simple.
- **C3:** complete articular fracture in which both metaphyseal and articular components are multifragmentary (complex).

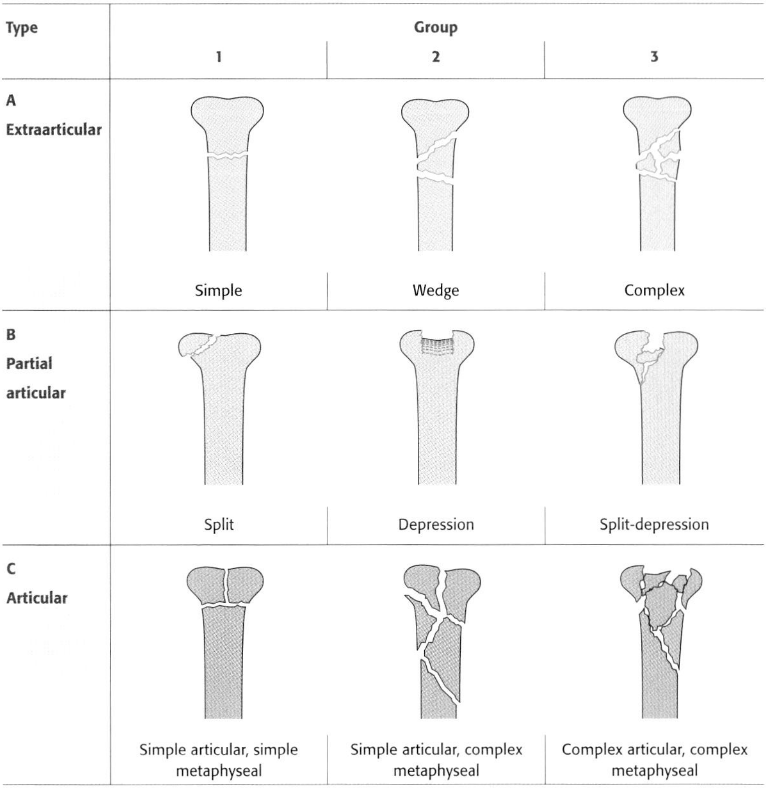

Type	Group		
	1	**2**	**3**
A **Extraarticular**			
	Simple	Wedge	Complex
B **Partial articular**			
	Split	Depression	Split-depression
C **Articular**			
	Simple articular, simple metaphyseal	Simple articular, complex metaphyseal	Complex articular, complex metaphyseal

Fig 1-5 Description of end-segment fractures.

Although the amount of displacement and angulation is not incorporated in the Müller AO Classification of fractures—long bones, it must be considered in the assessment and planning for management because displacement reflects the energy that was applied to the fracture zone.

1.4 Coding

The three types are labeled A, B, and C. Each type is divided into three groups: A1, A2, A3/B1, B2, B3/C1, C2, C3. Hence, there are nine groups.

Example: 33-C3

3	3	-	C	3
Femur	distal segment		complete articular	metaphyseal complex articular complex

Each group is further subdivided into three subgroups denoted by a number .1, .2, .3. Thus, there is for each segment 27 subgroups. The use of subgroups is largely confined to research. In clinical use most surgeons only classify down to the group level.

1.5 Soft-tissue injuries

An open fracture: If an injury of the soft tissue causes an open communication between a fracture or dislocation and the environment.

1.6 Gustilo classification of open fractures

This classification is the most commonly used in clinical practice. Although the size of the open wound may seem to be the main factor defining the degree of injury in the classification developed by Gustilo and Anderson, the fracture configuration and the degree of contamination also should be considered.

Type I: Wound smaller than 1 cm with little or no contamination, bone fragment perforates the skin (inside-out injury), simple fracture resulting from low-energy injury (Fig 1-6a–b).

Type II: Wound more than 1 cm with minor or no signs of contusion of the edges caused by direct trauma resulting in moderately comminuted fractures. Tension-free wound closure must be possible without skin graft or any kind of flaps (Fig 1-6c–d).

Type III: Extensive soft-tissue injury resulting from high-energy direct trauma. Usually the size of the wound is longer than 10 cm. The associated fracture is often comminuted or widely displaced. Regardless of wound size fractures caused by high-energy gun shot wounds, fractures sustained in a highly contaminated environment, and segmental fractures belong in this category (Fig 1-6e–f).

Type IIIA: Despite the extensive soft-tissue injury, the fractured bone can still be covered with adequate local soft tissue. The wound is covered by delayed primary closure or with a skin graft.

Type IIIB: Extensive soft-tissue loss with periosteal stripping is present; the bone cannot be covered with vital tissue and requires coverage by rotational or free-flap reconstruction.

Type IIIC: Any type of open fracture with accompanying arterial injury requiring repair.

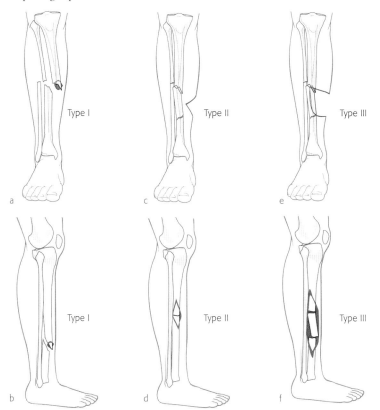

Fig 1-6a–f   Gustilo classification of fractures according to the severity of the complicating wound. A complex diaphyseal fracture which is a result of direct trauma may be related to a small open wound. These injuries should be classified as type III. Final decision on classification of an open fracture must be made only after thorough debridement and with the patient under general anesthesia.

1.7   AO soft-tissue grading system

The grading of the skin (integument) injury is done separately for open and closed fractures. IC indicates skin injury in closed fractures; IO, skin injury in open fractures.

IC 1	No evident skin lesion
IC 2	No skin laceration, but contusion
IC 3	Circumscribed degloving
IC 4	Extensive, closed degloving
IC 5	Necrosis from contusion

Table 1-1   AO soft-tissue classification: closed skin lesions (IC).

IO 1	Skin breakage from inside out
IO 2	Skin breakage from outside in <5 cm, contused edges
IO 3	Skin breakage from outside in >5 cm, increased contusion, devitalized edges
IO 4	Considerable, full-thickness contusion, abrasion, extensive open degloving, skin loss
IO 5	Extensive degloving

Table 1-2   AO soft-tissue classification: open skin lesions (IO).

Part I

2   Wound healing and fracture healing

2 Wound healing and fracture healing

2.1 Wound healing

A wound is a disruption of the normal anatomical structure of tissues as a result of direct or indirect trauma. Wound healing focuses on the recovery of the continuity of the tissues by remodeling the form while retaining their mechanical and functional characteristics.

The wound-healing process can be divided into stages which partly overlap each other. Characteristic inflammatory processes, all involving specific cellular reactions, play a role and occur in a fixed chronological sequence.

Depending on the nature of the wound and the treatment applied, two types of wound healing are distinguished:

- **Primary wound healing (sanatio per primam):** This healing occurs if the wound has sharp edges that are attached together (by stitches). The two edges adhere due to fibrin formation. Migration of epithelial cells starts within a few hours, so that the injury is bridged within a few days. Collagen fibers attach the edges of the wound together to ensure a quick recovery of continuity (Fig 2-1).
- **Secondary wound healing (sanatio per secundam):** This occurs if the wound edges are not opposed or tissue loss occurs. The wound is initially filled up with granulomatous tissue. Epithelization occurs starting from the wound edges (Fig 2-2).

2.2 Stages in wound healing

First stage
Duration: 5–7 days.
Characteristics: homeostasis and inflammatory reaction.
Homeostasis by:
- Vasoconstriction due to the elasticity and contractibility of the vessel wall
- Activation of the clotting mechanism

Because of a complex interaction among thrombocytes, clotting factors, and damaged vessel walls, cellular and humoral reactions occur.

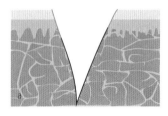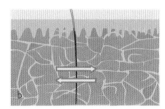

Fig 2-1a–b   Primary wound healing.

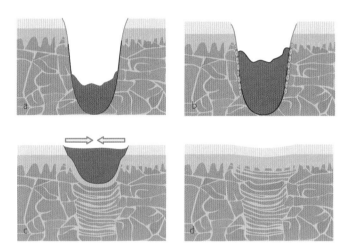

Fig 2-2a–d   Secondary wound healing illustrated step-by-step.
a–b Formation of granulation tissue; c maturation and conraction;
d epithelization followed by remodeling.

The coagulation cascade with thrombocyte aggregation and formation of fibrin (threads) leads to a homeostatic clot.

Inflammatory reaction caused by:

- Vasodilatation (starting within 5–10 minutes) with a slowing of the blood flow and stasis
- Exudation, fluid, and cells migrate through the permeable endothelial wall of the capillaries
- Chemotaxis and proliferation of granulocytes and monocytes
- Phagocytosis and lysis of the damaged tissue and bacteria
- Formation of endothelial cells and fibroblasts

Second stage

Duration: 1 to several weeks.

Characteristics: migration, proliferation, and angiogenesis.

Migration and proliferation of:

- Mesenchymal cells (fibroblasts) that mediate the production of connective tissue components, such as collagen, elastin, and ground substance, which determine the mechanical strength of the healing wound.

Angiogenesis by:

- Endothelial cells that build up a capillary network that gives the richly vascularized granulation tissue a gritty texture.

Third stage

Duration: several weeks to months.

Characteristics: maturation and contraction.

Maturation:

- The scar formation is completed and fibroblasts, macrophages, and capillaries disappear from the granulation tissue. The strength of the scar tissue increases because newly formed collagen fibers form a strong matrix. This process is controlled by the physiological load in the form of pressure and contraction forces.

Contraction:

- Fibroblasts causing puckering of the wound surface differentiate into myofibroblasts with contractile properties. This phenomenon particularly occurs in secondary wound healing and results in an open wound shrinking during the healing process, so that the area of injured skin that will eventually need to be bridged by epithelization is reduced.

End stage

Duration: several months to more than 1 year.

Characteristics: color change and remodeling.

Color change:

■ Capillaries disappear, hyperemia also decreases. This phenomenon makes a red and "fiery" new scar become paler.

Remodeling:

■ Return the original elasticity of the tissue by restoration of the collagen structure. The scar acquires its definite shape (width, hypertrophy, or keloid) and color (pale or pigmented).

2.3 Factors delaying wound healing

Local factors that delay wound healing are:

■ Infection
■ Tissue hypoxia
■ Foreign body
■ Radiation

General factors that delay wound healing are:

■ Malnutrition
■ Use of corticosteroids/NSAIDs
■ Chemotherapy
■ Diabetes mellitus
■ Dehydration
■ Heavy smoking

2.4 Fracture healing

A fracture is a disruption of the normal anatomical structure of bone tissue caused by direct or indirect trauma which is always associated with injury of the soft tissue (Fig 2-3). Fracture healing is focused on recovery of the bone integrity and with this the function of the affected part of the body.

Bone is the only tissue in the body that heals by replication of normal tissue as opposed to scar tissue formation. The conditions needed for this are adequate vascularization of bone fragments, presence of cells that can form new bone tissue, and sufficient mechanical stability of the fracture.

- Contact between the ends of the fracture is not essential.

Depending on the treatment used and the resulting stability and blood supply to the ends of the fractured bone, two forms of fracture healing are distinguished:
- **Direct (primary) fracture healing:** This occurs after rigid fixation (osteosynthesis) of perfectly aligned fracture ends (Fig 2-4). The fracture ends are joined together by outgrowths from the many haversian canals from one bone fragment to the other. Haversian canals form osteons that contain osteoclasts in the "head" which connect up with the bone opposite to allow multiple osteoblasts to start forming new bone in these canals (Fig 2-5). Endosteal and periosteal callus formation does not occur. The bone ends are closely in contact and are compressed by the treatment given. Primary fracture healing is not visible on x-rays, and is slower than secondary healing.
- **Indirect (secondary) fracture healing:** This occurs in the same way as wound healing, namely in stages which partly overlap each other. Callus formation is part of this healing process.

First stage
Duration: 1–3 days.
Characteristics: fracture hematoma and inflammatory reaction (Fig 2-6a).
Fracture hematoma:
- Rupture of blood vessels in the bone and surrounding soft tissue

Inflammatory reaction:
- Vasodilatation with slowing of blood flow and stasis
- Proliferation of granulocytes, macrophages, and monocytes derived from the bloodstream
- Proliferation of omnipotent mesenchymal stem cells (precursors of fibroblasts, osteoblasts, and osteoclasts) from the periosteum and the endosteum

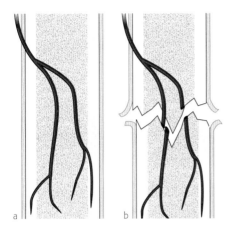

Fig 2-3a–b Tissue structures involved in a fracture.

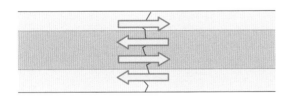

Fig 2-4 Osteons that cross over the fracture split and bridge the bone.

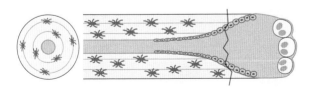

Fig 2-5 Osteon with osteoclasts in the head and osteoblasts in the tail.

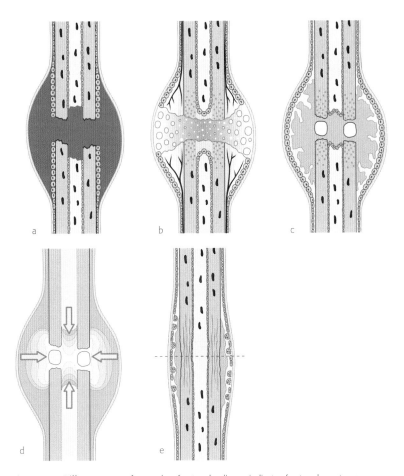

Fig 2-6a–e   Different stages of secondary fracture healing: a indicates fracture hematoma;
b granulation formation with invasion by fibroblasts and ingrowth of blood vessels; c fibrous callus,
osteoblast activity; d callus; e remodeling and complete healing.

Second stage

Duration: 3 weeks.

Characteristic: granulation formation (Fig 2-6b).

- **Fibroblasts and endothelial cells:** These form a network of fibrin, collagen fibers, and many capillaries in the hematoma through which the first connection between parts of the fracture is made. As the tissue is not yet mineralized, this is known as soft callus or osteoid; it is not visible on x-rays.

- **Osteoblasts:** These cells start the actual bone formation while the osteoclasts break down the necrotic fracture ends. Both endosteal and periosteal callus formation occur.

Third stage

Duration: 2–4 weeks.

Characteristic: osseous callus formation (Fig 2-6c–d).

- Deposition of hydroxyapatite in the ground substance between the fibrous networks which results in a hardening of the callus mass. As the amount of minerals increases in the callus, it becomes visible on an x-ray. When the callus becomes so hard that there is no longer any movement possible between parts of the fracture, on physiological loading clinical consolidation has been reached.

End stage

Duration: months to years.

Characteristic: remodeling (Fig 2-6e).

- Osteoclasts break down the newly formed callus and osteoblasts build up new bone. The formation of this lamellar bone is controlled by physiological load. The greater the load the more bone is deposited. In this period excess callus is reabsorbed and a new medullary cavity is created. Radiographic consolidation is then achieved. The remodeling process occurs according to Wolff law, namely that bone is produced at sites where the mechanical load is high and broken down where the bone is not or only slightly under stress (Fig 2-6e).

2.5   Factors delaying fracture healing

Local factors that delay fracture healing are:
- Infection
- Insufficient vascularization because of trauma or surgery
- Insufficient mechanical stability
- Radiation

General factors that delay fracture healing are:
- Use of corticosteroids/NSAIDs
- Chemotherapy
- Heavy smoking

■ Osteoporosis does not have a profound negative effect on fracture healing.

2.6   Ways to promote fracture healing

The following measures can promote fracture healing:
- Stabilization by means of osteosynthesis
- Covering any soft-tissue defect with a vascularized tissue transplant
- Decortication
- Autologous bone transplant
- Electromagnetic stimulation
- Growth factors, including BMP (bone morphogenic protein)
- Ultrasound
- Functional loading

3   Principles of fracture treatment

3 Principles of fracture treatment

3.1 Introduction

The aim of fracture treatment is to restore function in the broadest sense of the word, not only the load-bearing ability of the affected bone and the mobility of the surrounding joints but also getting patients to return to activities of daily living, such as work, hobbies, and exercise.

3.2 Basics of fracture treatment

The cornerstones of fracture treatment are:
- Reduction
- Immobilization
- Rehabilitation

Reduction
A distinction is made between nonanatomical and anatomical reduction.

Nonanatomical reduction (functional reduction)
Children: Used for extraarticular fractures. Because of remodeling potential in children most deviations in anatomical position (except for rotation) will be corrected spontaneously. The degree of remodeling depends on a child's age.
Adults: Used in fractures of the humeral shaft; deviations in anatomical position are well tolerated cosmetically and functionally. Used in femoral and tibial shaft fractures; length, rotation, and axis should be normal, slight lateral displacement is acceptable (valgus).

Anatomical reduction
Children: Used for some epiphyseal fractures; those are intraarticular fractures (Salter-Harris types III and IV). If reduction is not perfect a fracture gap will be left. A persistent fracture gap fills with callus which forms a bridge between the epiphysis and the metaphysis. Consequently, the growth plate is closed which can result in local epiphyseodesis and growth arrest.
Adults: Used for intraarticular fractures. A failure to achieve anatomical reduction leads to joint incongruity and ultimately arthrosis. Reduction can be obtained either by opening the fracture site by a surgical approach and mani-

pulating the fracture fragments directly—direct reduction, or by applying a force distant from the fracture site (usually traction) and achieving reduction by indirect means—indirect reduction. Anatomical reduction is usually obtained by direct (open) reduction. Direct reduction is potentially more traumatic, particularly regarding blood supply to the fracture.

Immobilization

The following options are available:

- Rigid: use plates and screws, eg, in osteosynthesis of talus fracture to improve revascularization of the talar head.
- Semirigid: use intramedullary nails; most fractures in cortical bone. Damage to the blood supply is limited.
- Nonrigid: traction, plaster, brace; use K-wires for distal radial fractures.
- No immobilization is effective in clavicular fractures, rib fractures, and pubic bone fractures.

Rehabilitation

The aim of rehabilitation is to promote functional recovery and to prevent fracture disease.

Fracture disease is the complex of signs and symptoms that occurs after a fracture and the related soft-tissue injury. It is closely associated with treatment involving prolonged immobilization of joints and muscles and nonweight bearing.

- Etiology: inactivity, immobilization, nonweight-bearing status
- Pathology: muscular atrophy, circulatory dysfunction bone atrophy, and joint stiffness
- Treatment: physiotherapy, such as isotonic or isometric muscle training (in a plaster cast). Prevention by early mobilization and weight-bearing exercises is the best therapy.

3.3 Conservative treatment

Conservative treatment involves functional treatment or closed (noninvasive) immobilization with or without closed reduction.

Indications

Nondisplaced fractures and fractures when displacement is accepted, such as:

- Clavicular, scapular, or rib fractures
- Most stable vertebral and pelvic fractures
- Most extraarticular fractures in children: the remodeling potential enables the anatomy to recover
- Displaced extraarticular fractures when the anatomical position can be maintained after reduction by closed (external) immobilization, eg, fractures of the wrist, hand, or lower leg

Procedures

The following options are available:

- Functional treatment: eg, with clavicular fractures, rib fractures, and pubic bone fractures—analgesia and early active mobilization when pain allows.
- Bed rest: this is no longer acceptable because of potential problems like pneumonia, thrombosis, and decubitus. Stable vertebral fractures receive a functional treatment with early mobilization.
- Reduction by manipulation followed by immobilization in a plaster cast, eg, in fractures of the wrist, hand, and lower leg, especially in children.
- Traction: skin traction (tape), skeletal traction (K-wires or Steinmann pin), eg, in shaft fractures in children. Traction is rarely indicated in adults except as a temporary measure, ie, use of modified Thomas splints for femoral shaft fractures before emergency surgery (Figs 3-1, 3-2).
- Reduction by manipulation followed by immobilization: eg, in supracondylar humeral fractures in children with collar and cuff immobilization.
- Functional brace, usually as a cylinder of thermoplastic or semirigid material with which a broken long bone is partially immobilized leaving adjoining joints free, eg, in fractures of the humeral and tibial shaft. Functional braces cannot prevent shortening, so should only be used in fractures where the fracture pattern is such that shortening will not occur, ie, reduced simple transverse fractures (Fig 3-3).

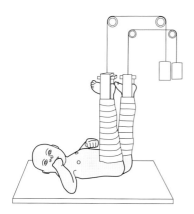

Fig 3-1 Fracture of the femoral shaft in a child treated with traction according to Bryant.

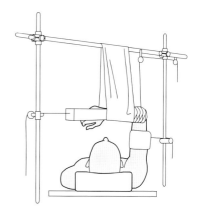

Fig 3-2 Supracondylar humoral fracture treated with olecranon traction.

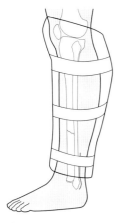

Fig 3-3 Fracture of the lower leg treated with a functional brace.

Casting

- Avoid local pressure during hardening of the plaster cast to prevent local skin ischemia and thus necrosis.
- Ensure joints that do not need to be immobilized can move freely.
- Ensure padding of prominent bone with cotton or synthetic wool, eg, fibula head, ankle joint (lateral and medial malleoli).
- Immobilize a new fracture with a splint or in a padded, split cast because the injured extremity can swell up. Swelling in the presence of a full cast may cause compartment syndrome.
- Elevate the immobilized extremity (see chapter 14 "Compartment syndrome and posttraumatic dystrophy").
- Monitor for disorders of the peripheral circulation, motor system, and sensibility in the immobilized extremity after a new injury. Also check carefully for increasing pain, which is the cardinal sign of compartment syndrome.

3.4   Surgical treatment

Surgical treatment involves open or closed reduction of the fracture followed by immobilization using internal or external fixation.

Indications

Fractures for which conservative treatment is not indicated are:

- Open fractures (with an open connection between the fracture and the environment); stabilization of the fracture limits the risk of infection.
- Displaced intraarticular fractures; nonanatomical reduction results in incongruity which can lead to posttraumatic arthrosis, especially in the lower extremity bearing the greatest load.
- Avulsion fractures caused by traction to a muscle/tendon complex; without fixation, diastasis will persist with a great risk of pseudarthrosis (humerus epicondylus, olecranon, patella).
- All femoral shaft fractures.

Methods

A distinction is made between internal and external fixation.

Internal fixation: the immobilizing implant is under the skin (Figs 3-4, 3-5).

External fixation: the immobilizing material is almost completely secured outside the skin (Fig 3-6). With this method the risk of infection of the fracture area is minimal; therefore, it is especially used in serious open fractures, in fractures with serious accompanying soft-tissues injuries, or if an infection occurs in the course of fracture treatment. The disadvantage of this method is the risk of pin-track infection. Meticulous care of the pins is vital.

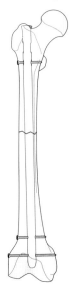

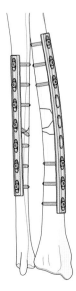

Fig 3-4   Femoral shaft fracture with a locked intramedullary nail.

Fig 3-5   Fracture of the lower arm treated with plates and screws.

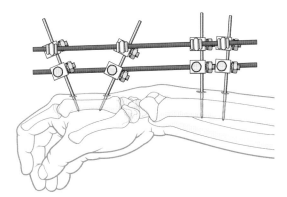

Fig 3-6   Distal radial fracture treated with external fixation.

Procedures

The following options are available:

■   Closed reduction and percutaneous internal fixation using K-wires (Fig 3-7a) or screws: eg, proximal humerus, distal radius. Radial fractures normally need additional cast immobilization.

■   Closed reduction and intramedullary fixation: eg, locking nail in femur or tibia

■   Closed reduction and internal fixation: eg, distal radius or tibia

■   Open reduction and internal fixation: eg, plate on ulna and/or radius

■   Combination of internal and external fixation: eg, fractures of the tibial plateau or of the distal tibial joint area (pilon fracture) with extension to the tibial shaft. Due to the vulnerable soft-tissue situation around the knee and ankle, internal fixation is limited to reconstruction of the joint area, if necessary with cancellous bone screws inserted percutaneously; the rest of the fracture area is immobilized with external fixation (Fig 3-7b).

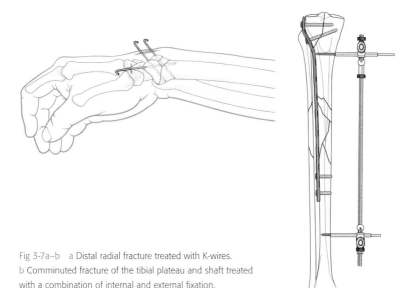

Fig 3-7a–b   a Distal radial fracture treated with K-wires.
b Comminuted fracture of the tibial plateau and shaft treated with a combination of internal and external fixation.

Soft tissue

Be aware of open and closed soft-tissue injuries, eg, decollement, compartment syndrome.

Do not close soft tissue at the end of operation if tension would occur. Leave the wound open and close it with artificial skin or vacuum sealing.

■ If administered preoperatively, antimicrobial prophylaxis reduces the risk of wound infection after surgical treatment of fractures. In open fractures prophylaxis should be given as soon as possible.

Timing

Immediately after injury, the condition of the soft tissue is most favorable for surgical treatment. If treatment is delayed, the limb must be elevated and the fracture should be temporarily immobilized in a plaster cast or by traction until the swelling has decreased and soft tissues have improved. In severe soft-tissue injuries associated with high-energy trauma, temporary immobilization is often best achieved by application of an external fixator. Pins are inserted into the bone above and below the zone of injury—spanning external fixator.

Mechanical function of implants

A distinction is made between rigid implants achieving compression and splints which permit a slight degree of movement at the fracture site. Implants can obtain compression at a fracture site in various ways.

■ A screw can be inserted across the fracture site so as to achieve compression—the interfragmentary screw. Compression using the interfragmentary screw can either be achieved by the design of the screw where the thread is only on the distal far end, or any screw can achieve compression providing the proximal (near cortex) is overdrilled so the screw slides through the hole with only its distal screw thread gripping the far cortex (Fig 3-8).

■ In those bones which are eccentrically loaded, such as the femur, one cortex is under tension and the other under compressive forces when the bone is subjected to physiological load. If a plate is applied to the tension side of the bone, the tension forces are converted to compression forces on the opposite cortex when the bone is under physiological load (Fig 3-9).

■ Wire can be inserted on either side of the fracture site, eg, in fractures of the olecranon and patella, so that when the wire is tightened compression is applied to the fracture site (Fig 3-10).

■ Certain fractures will only displace in one direction when subjected to physiological load. If a plate is applied to resist this motion then the fracture will come under compressive forces when physiological loading is applied—buttress plate (Fig 3-11).

■ Splints can be internal or external to the body. Internal splinting includes intramedullary nailing where the implant lies in the medulla (Fig 3-12). Plates can also be applied without compression and when a plate is used in this way—a bridge plate—it acts as a splint and not a compression device. If applied as a wave plate, bone grafting below the plate is also possible (Fig 3-13). External splintage: Splinting of a fracture site can also be achieved using external fixation (Fig 3-14).

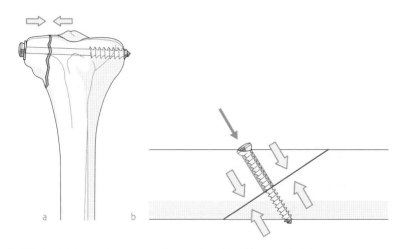

Fig 3-8a–b   Interfragmentary screws. a Compression achieved by screw design.
b Compression achieved by overdrilling the near cortex.

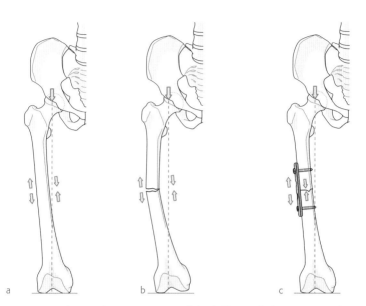

Fig 3-9a–c   a The intact femur is an eccentrically loaded bone with distraction or tensile forces laterally and compression on the medial side. In case of fracture: b The lateral fracture gap will open, whereas the medial will be compressed. c If a lateral plate is placed alongside the linea aspera of the femur, it will be under tension when loaded; thus compressing the fracture gap, provided there is bone contact medially.

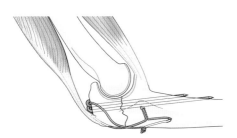

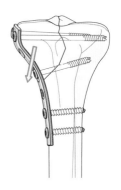

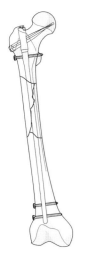

Fig 3-10   Tension band wire.

Fig 3-11   Buttress plate. Fracture will displace under load in direction shown by arrow. Plate resists this displacement.

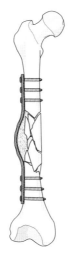

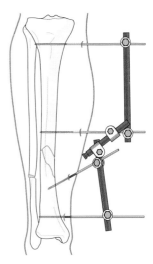

Fig 3-12   Intramedullary locking nail.

Fig 3-13   Wave plate allowing for grafting of lateral defect.

Fig 3-14   External fixation.

Preoperative care

The preoperative care consists of:

- History of mechanism of injury—high or low energy.

  - Think about pathological fractures if force is minimal.

- Physical examination that is especially focused on diagnosing possible accompanying neurovascular injuries.
- Assessment of soft-tissue injury to determine the timing of surgery; in open fractures, surgery is undertaken within a few hours. If severe soft-tissue swelling exists, surgery should be delayed to allow recovery of the soft tissue. Short-term immobilization of the fracture is usually achieved by the use of a spanning external fixator.
- Measuring tissue pressure when compartment syndrome is suspected, eg, in fractures of the lower leg (see chapter 14 "Compartment syndrome and posttraumatic dystrophy").
- Taking adequate x-rays; in diaphyseal fractures both adjoining joints should be visible.
- Temporary splinting of the affected limb to reduce pain.
- Elevating the affected limb to reduce swelling.
- Thrombosis prophylaxis.
- Analgesia.
- Antibiotic prohylaxis for open fractures as soon as possible and preoperatively for all closed fractures to be treated surgically.

Follow-up care

The follow-up care consists of:

- A temporary splint to reduce pain, swelling, and tendency to adopt an abnormal position of function (eg, equinus position of ankle).
- Elevating the limb to reduce swelling.
- Early active mobilization in patients treated by fixation. Achieving stability by osteosynthesis so that external immobilization (in a plaster cast or by traction) is not necessary and the patient can start exercising directly after the operation is vital. Whether exercises are weight bearing or not depends on type and quality of the osteosynthesis.
- A plaster cast is used if sufficient stability is not achieved after osteosynthesis to allow weight bearing (eg, after osteosynthesis of an ankle fracture).
- Removing implants if they cause symptoms.

Local postoperative complications

The following local postoperative complications can occur:

- Hematoma in the operated area. In case of persistent leakage of blood through the wound, re-exploration under sterile conditions (in the operating room) is indicated; the treatment consists of irrigation, debridement, and closing the wound again around a suction drain.
- Infected hematoma: exploratory surgery under sterile conditions, irrigation, debridement, and local and systemic antibiotic treatment.

Advantages and disadvantages of conservative and surgical treatment

Advantages and disadvantages exist to both treatment options regarding risk of infection, fracture disease, and costs. The major disadvantage of surgical treatment is infection.

The risk of infection is on average 1–2% after surgical treatment of closed fractures. Risk factors are old age, malnutrition, diabetes, smoking, open fractures and/or soft-tissue injuries, contamination, inadequate surgical technique, long duration of the operation, and hematoma formation.

Symptoms of fracture disease can be prevented or reduced by early active mobilization and weight bearing, if possible, of the affected limb directly after surgery.

Costs of implants used in fracture surgery are compensated by savings in nursing care costs. Early active mobilization shortens the duration of the disability. Overall surgical treatment normally reduces the total cost of the injury—hospital and possible disability costs.

3.5   Fractures in children

A pediatric fracture is a broken bone with open epiphyseal growth plates in a child or young adolescent.

Anatomy and (patho)physiology

Children's bones consist of the diaphysis which is surrounded by a strong and well-vascularized periosteum with an epiphysis (growth plates) at both ends. The growth plate and the periosteum are responsible for lengthening and thickening of the bone, respectively. In children, because of functional loading, there is a continual process of building up and breaking down of bone mass.

The specific properties of children's bones explain the differences in fracture healing between children and adults. The thick periosteum promotes callus formation and speeds up fracture healing. Pseudarthrosis seldom occurs in children. Cosmetic and functional deformities of the bone are corrected spontaneously by asymmetric thickening and lengthening of the bone. Asymmetric pressure to the growth plate corrects axial deviation by differentially stimulating the epiphyseal cells on the "short" side. Shortening of the bone is corrected by stimulation of the epiphyseal plate, probably because of an increased blood supply to the fracture area. The younger a child is the greater the potential to spontaneously correct the axis and length (Fig 3-15).

■ There is little correction of rotational malunion.

The growth plate is a delicate structure and if damaged can lead to serious growth arrest. The growth plate consists of cartilage cells (chondrocytes) from the actual growth zone (basal epidermis). Dividing chondrocytes migrate in the direction of the shaft, while differentiating and ossifying (Fig 3-16). A fracture through this ossifying zone does not disturb growth because the basal epidermis itself is spared. A fracture that runs through the growth area is known as an epiphyseal fracture. If not treated correctly, there is a high risk of growth arrest.

Classification

According to the Salter-Harris classification, five types of injuries of the epiphysis plate occur:

Type I   Fracture through zone of ossification (Fig 3-17a)
Type II   Fracture through zone of ossification with metaphyseal fragment (Fig 3-17b)
Type III   Epiphyseal fracture (Fig 3-17c)
Type IV   Epiphyseal fracture extending to the metaphysis (Fig 3-17d)
Type V   Compression of the growth plate (Fig 3-17e)

Types I and II have a favorable prognosis. In types III, IV, and V, there is a risk of growth arrest because the basal epithelium is damaged. In epiphyseal fractures anatomical reduction, usually with surgical fixation, is needed to prevent growth arrest (Figs 3-18, 3-19).

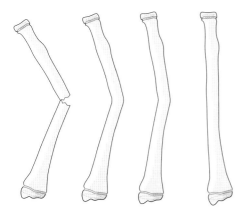

Fig 3-15   Remodeling of shaft fracture in a child.

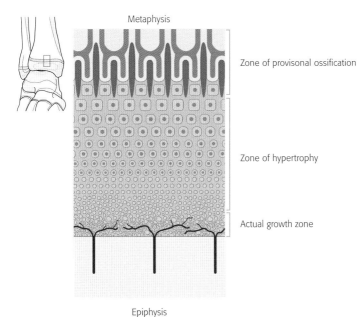

Metaphysis

Zone of provisonal ossification

Zone of hypertrophy

Actual growth zone

Epiphysis

Fig 3-16   Illustration of the epiphyseal (growth) plate.

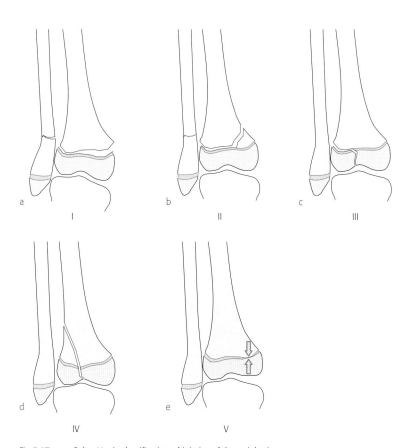

Fig 3-17a–e   Salter-Harris classification of injuries of the epiphysis.

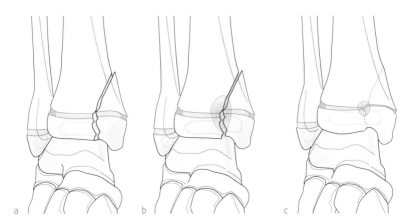

Fig 3-18a–c   Because of callus formation, growth arrest occurs between the epiphysis and meta-physis after a type IV injury.

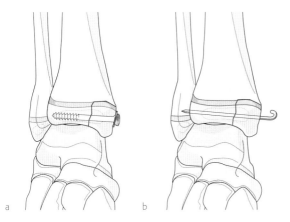

Fig 3-19a–b   Examples of internal fixation after anatomical reduction of a type III injury according to the Salter-Harris classification.

Diagnostics

Clinical examination is important because it is not always possible to take a reliable case history in children. A thorough knowledge of the ossification process is required to evaluate plain x-rays adequately. If it is not possible to decide whether there is a fracture, a magnetic resonance imaging (MRI) scan is required.

In infants ultrasound is indicated in shoulder, elbow, or hip injuries when a fracture is not visible on plain x-rays (birth trauma, dislocation, or epiphysiolysis). If in doubt, a computed tomographic (CT) scan or MRI is sometimes indicated (pelvis, vertebral column). In young patients arthrography is seldom used.

Treatment

The goal of treatment is to prevent sequelae such as contractures, excessive growth, growth arrest, secondary axis deviation, and joint incongruity. In a child long-term immobilization of the limbs does not have negative effect on the joints; posttraumatic dystrophy seldom occurs. Conservative treatment is indicated in most extraarticular fractures. This consists of careful reduction (preferably only once) under narcosis and immobilization in a plaster cast or traction bandage, depending on the stability achieved.

Up until 2 years before the end of the growth period (girls about 13 years, boys about 15 years), the aim is healing with some shortening; slight lateral displacement and axis deviation may be accepted.

- Rotational abnormalities hardly spontaneously correct with growth and should be avoided.

Strong indications for operative treatment in children are:

- Epiphyseal fractures: if not reduced well, with a risk of growth arrest and joint incongruity.
- Avulsion and dislocated fractures (epicondylus, olecranon, patella).
- Fractures with vascular injury and/or manifest or threatened compartment syndrome.
- Fractures with associated joint dislocation: eg, Monteggia and Galeazzi fractures.
- A forearm fracture that has been insufficiently reduced (angulation ≥10°) or is unstable.
- Unstable injuries to vertebrae.

Relative indications for operative treatment are:
- Fractures of the femoral shaft (shorter hospitalization)
- Difficulty in immobilizing a fracture close to a joint
- Fractures in polytrauma and/or coma patients
- Ligament and muscle avulsion with risk of growth disturbance or pseudarthrosis, eg, elbow, knee

The follow-up treatment for conservative and surgical therapy is in principle the same and consists of:
- Close monitoring of circulation and nerve function
- Replacing the cast about 2–3 weeks after reduction; if the fracture is considered to be sufficiently stable because of fibrous callus formation, this can be done without narcosis
- Removing the osteosynthesis material after a few weeks or months depending on fracture healing

Duration of treatment

To calculate the healing time of shaft fractures (in weeks) the following rule is used: age in years + 1. For example: the healing time of a 3-year-old child is $3 + 1 = 4$ weeks. Fractures of the upper limb heal faster than fractures of the lower limb.

- Osteosynthesis increases the mobility of a child but does not speed up the healing time of a fracture. Osteosynthesis leads to shorter hospitalization, thus earlier reintegration into the family.

Prognosis

Shaft fractures normally heal without any problems. Children with epiphyseal fractures should be followed up for at least 1 year.

- The child's parents/guardians should be informed about the risk of growth disturbance.

3.6 Pathological fractures

A pathological fracture is a fracture, generally resulting from minimal trauma, occurring in a bone that has been weakened by a systemic or local abnormality. The incidence of tumor is less than 1% of all fractures. However, osteoporosis accounts for more than 50% of fractures in some countries.

Causes

Local causes of pathological fractures are:

- Tumors (metastasis, 50%)
- Osteomyelitis
- Radionecrosis

General causes of pathological fractures are:

- Osteoporosis
- Osteogenesis imperfecta
- Renal osteodystrophy
- Paget disease

Tumors

Benign tumors include:

- Juvenile bone cyst
- Aneurysmatic bone cyst
- Giant cell tumor
- Enchondroma

The diagnosis is made based on the x-ray and a biopsy specimen. Depending on the type, localization, and size of the tumor, the following therapeutic options are possible:

- Local injection with corticosteroids (in juvenile bone cyst)
- Small lesions can heal together with the fracture
- Sometimes local resection with cryotherapy, filled with bone graft

Malignant tumors include:

- Ewing sarcoma
- Chrondosarcoma
- Osteosarcoma

■ Always consider the possibility of a primary malignant bone tumor with pathological fractures.

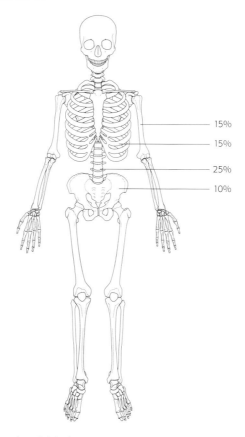

Fig 3-20   Most common sites of skeletal metastases.

A diagnosis is made based on the x-rays (Ewing sarcoma can resemble osteomyelitis because of fever, leukocytosis, and few bone abnormalities on original x-rays). Perform a CT scan, MRI, and skeletal scintigraphy, if necessary, and biopsy examination. A biopsy should not be performed until after the staging of the tumor and consultations with the national expert committees, preferably in the center where the therapy will take place.

Most malignant tumors involving bone are secondary. A diagnosis of metastases is based on the clinical presentation. The most common sites are vertebrae, pelvis, femur, humerus, ribs, and skull. Examples of malignant tumors that metastasize to the skeleton are (Fig 3-20):

- Breast carcinoma
- Lung carcinoma
- Prostate carcinoma
- Renal cell carcinoma (Grawitz tumor)
- Thyroid carcinoma
- With improved care of gastrointestinal tumors, bone metastases from these tumors are becoming more common

With metastases, the primary tumor is usually known; in cases when this is not so, the primary tumor is generally a lung carcinoma or renal cell carcinoma (Grawitz tumor). Pain is the first sign; it sometimes takes weeks before the x-ray shows any abnormalities. The pain does not respond well to analgesics. Multiple bone metastases cause hypercalcemia. Physical examination does not always show abnormalities either.

Metastases give a variable characteristic picture on x-ray with radiolucence, destruction, and sometimes osteoblastic reactive bone (prostate, breast) is seen. A bone scan can give a positive result if the overview x-ray is still negative and also provides information on the whole skeleton.

- Always take an x-ray of the whole bone from joint-to-joint to identify metastases elsewhere in the bone.

- Always consider the possibility of a primary bone tumor when diagnosing skeletal metastases with an as yet unknown primary tumor.

Treatment

The aim of treatment in pathological fractures is:
- For metastases: pain relief to facilitate nursing and increase mobility.
- For benign tumors and some primary bone tumors: healing.

Therapeutic options are:
- Radiotherapy for pathological fractures of the upper extremities caused by a metastasis: eg, breast.

■ Surgical treatment with intramedullary fixation (Fig 3-21), plate osteo-synthesis, with or without cement (Fig 3-22), or insertion of prosthesis (Fig 3-23) (hip), aiming at achieving a weight-bearing status.

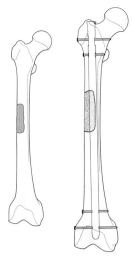

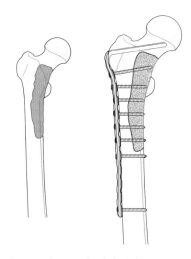

Fig 3-21 Threatened pathological fracture of the femur treated with locked medullary nail.

Fig 3-22 Threatened pathological fracture of the femur treated with a condylar blade plate and bone cement.

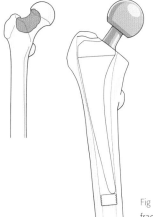

Fig 3-23 Threatened pathological femoral neck fracture treated with a hip prosthesis.

Treatment for threatened pathological fractures aims at actually preventing a pathological fracture.

Indications for prophylactic surgical treatment are:
- Pain that responds inadequately to other therapies
- Threatened paraplegia with an adequate life expectancy
- Osteolytic nidus affecting more than 50% of the circumference of the cortex on CT scan
- Proximal femur

  - In general, a life expectancy of at least 6 weeks is a condition for surgery.

3.7   Fatigue fractures

Fatigue fractures occur as a result of excessive and/or persistent load. Examples of fatigue fractures are:
- Fibula/tibia shaft (in endurance exercise—shin splints)
- Metatarsal bone II (march fracture in endurance exercise, Fig 3-24)
- Spinous process of C7—clay shoveller's neck
- Rib(s) because of chronic coughing
- Femur (because of prednisone use and/or severe osteoporosis)

The clinical presentation consists of sudden pain after intensive activities or exercise. On physical examination local pain on palpation is found, sometimes accompanied by axial pain with some swelling. In the early stages no abnormalities are seen on x-ray. After a few weeks the fracture line becomes visible due to osteolysis. Callus also becomes visible and is usually hypertrophic. A diagnosis of fatigue fracture can be made early by skeletal scintigraphy and MRI. The therapy consists of relieving the load and rest; immobilization is not essential. The healing time may be several months. The prognosis is excellent but recurrence is a major problem in elite athletes.

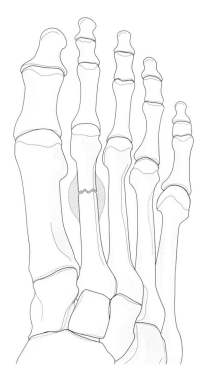

Fig 3-24   Fatigue fracture of the metatarsal bone II. After a few weeks the fracture line and callus become visible.

4 Polytrauma patients

4 Polytrauma patients

4.1 Introduction

Polytrauma patients have:
- Injuries involving more than one organ system.
- An Injury Severity Score (ISS) of ≥ 18. The ISS is calculated using a simple formula based on the sum of the severity of individual injuries to the six organ systems: central nervous system, thorax, abdomen, limbs, soft tissues, and circulation (see Table 4-1).

Note:
- About 70% of polytrauma patients have injuries to the skeletal system.
- The mortality rate increases with a higher ISS score, and increasing age.
- A multidisciplinary approach is needed for patients suffering multiple organ system injuries.

4.2 Emergency measures, diagnostics, and management

The initial diagnosis and management of polytrauma patients can be divided into four phases.

4.3 First phase (0–1 hour)

Emergency measures should be carried out systematically. The advanced trauma life support (ATLS) protocol provides a structured, systematic approach to the initial diagnosis and management of a polytrauma patient. The first hour after injury is known as the golden hour. The patient's chance of survival is frequently determined by the ability of medical personnel to identify and treat immediate life-threatening conditions in the first hour following injury.

The ATLS protocol dictates that examination and resuscitation be carried out in a structured fashion, following five steps from A to E.

A—airway

Establish and maintain an open airway, while controlling the cervical spine to prevent secondary spinal injury.

Cervical spine control and protection can be maintained during intubation by stabilizing the head and neck with light traction. Intubation can be safely performed before x-ray evaluation of the cervical spine if required, providing gentle traction is applied.

B—breathing

Provide supplemental oxygen therapy.

If spontaneous respiration is inadequate, the patient should receive mechanical ventilation.

Treat life-threatening thoracic injuries such as tension pneumothorax with immediate decompression.

C—circulation

Control active external hemorrhage with application of direct pressure to the bleeding site.

Rapidly identify potential sites of internal hemorrhage.

Restore normal circulation by increasing intravascular volume with the initial infusion of 2 liters of normal saline.

D—disability

Evaluate the patient's neurological status and assign a grade of injury according to the Glasgow Coma Scale.

E—exposure

Undress the patient completely to examine the entire body for signs and symptoms of injury.

During the process of exposure, be aware of the temperature of the environment and keep the patient warm and limit exposure time to prevent a decrease in body temperature.

Once the initial A to E survey has been performed and vital signs stabilized, a more detailed secondary survey should be done to fully identify the extent of injuries to all organ systems. Based on this examination, additional x-rays and diagnostic studies are performed to further identify all injuries. Injured extremities should be splinted during the secondary survey.

Specific injuries that need to be addressed in the golden hour include:
- Airway obstruction
- Tension pneumothorax
- Pneumothorax
- Hemothorax
- Flail chest
- Cardiac tamponade
- Severe hemorrhage (chest, abdomen, pelvis, multiple fractures)
- Coma (intracranial hemorrhage)
- Paraplegia

> ■ A polytrauma patient's condition can change without warning. The ABC portion of the examination needs to be repeated frequently to prevent deterioration and death.

Identification and management of selected specific injuries in the golden hour

Spinal column and spinal cord injury
The patient's head and neck must be immobilized with a rigid cervical collar and sandbags. The thoracic and lumbar spine should be protected with a backboard. Spinal precautions should be maintained until the cervical and thoracolumbar spine has been examined clinically and x-rayed for injury. If spinal precautions need to be maintained beyond the initial period or resuscitation, cervical spine immobilization should be maintained in the form of a cervical collar but the patient should be removed from the backboard to prevent pressure sores, and log-rolling precautions initiated to prevent additional spinal column injury.

X-rays

Cervical spine x-rays should be obtained from all polytrauma patients and should include the AP, lateral, and odontoid views. The lateral x-ray needs to extend and visualize the C7/T1 junction. X-rays should be evaluated for both soft-tissue and bone abnormalities. The prevertebral area should be assessed for soft-tissue swelling. The alignment of the cervical spine should be evaluated, and the vertebral bodies and other osseous structures should be reviewed for fracture.

X-rays of the thoracic and lumbar spine should be obtained based on clinical examination and suspicion of injury. Injuries of the thoracolumbar spine usually occur at the junction of the thoracic and lumbar vertebrae. X-rays need to demonstrate this area clearly, and should be specifically directed to this area.

■ 40% of spinal cord injuries occur in the area of the cervical thoracic junction (C6, C7, and T1), an area that is difficult to view adequately on x-rays.
■ 20% of patients with a spinal column injury at one level will have an injury at another level.

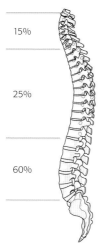

15%

25%

60%

Fig 4-1 Distribution of vertebral fractures at different spinal levels.

Signs and symptoms of spinal cord injuries can be:
- Loss of sensation (Fig 4-2)
- Muscle weakness or paralysis
- Reduced tone of the anal sphincter muscle
- Neurogenic shock
- Hypotension and bradycardia
- Priapism

■ Spinal cord injury level needs to be documented with a careful sensory and motor examination, so a baseline level of injury can be established if possible.

■ With increasing neurological deficit, further diagnostic studies and stabilization should be performed urgently. This might include realignment of the spinal column and decompression of the spinal cord.

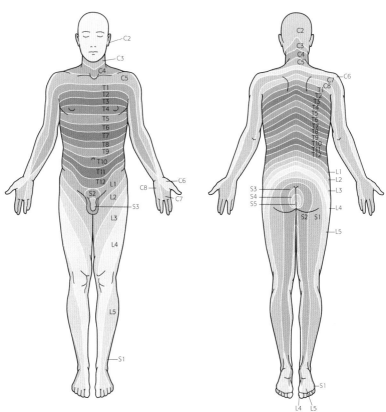

Fig 4-2a–b   Spinal sensory levels in relation to
the level on the spinothalamic tract.

Pelvic fractures

Significant blood loss can occur in patients with a mechanically unstable pelvic ring injury. Unexplained hypovolemic shock despite adequate infusion therapy may be seen.

In most cases pelvic hemorrhage is the result of bleeding from the sacral venous plexus, or fractured bone surfaces. Bleeding from these sources can be controlled by limiting pelvic motion to allow clot formation, and by reducing the pelvic volume to allow tamponade of the pelvic hematoma. Limitation of pelvic motion and reduction of pelvic volume can be achieved in injuries with a pelvic binder or anterior-based external fixator. Alternatively resuscitation clamp (C-clamp) placed in the iliac crest may be used. These measures are part of the resuscitation process and are generally undertaken in the emergency department or operating room (Figs 4-3, 4-4, and 4-5).

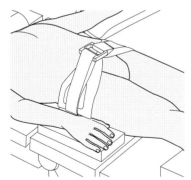

Fig 4-3   Unstable anterior pelvic ring disruption treated with pelvic binder.

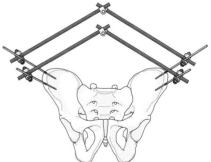

Fig 4-4   Unstable anterior pelvic ring disruption stabilized with anterior external fixator.

■ Persistent blood loss associated with an unstable pelvic fracture is only of arterial origin in approximately 10% of cases. The indication for pelvic angiography with an attempt at embolization is limited and should only be considered in patients with persistent blood loss despite mechanical stabilization and adequate fluid resuscitation.

Pelvic fractures can be associated with injuries to the genitourinary tract, rectum, vagina, and are occasionally open to the floor of perineum. Unrecognized and undertreated open pelvic fractures can result in a rapid septic-associated death. Inspection of the perineum and manual rectal and vaginal examinations are required in all pelvic fracture evaluations.

■ A diverting colostomy should be performed in patients with rectal and perineal injuries associated with pelvic fractures.

The following findings on examination are suggestive of a urethral injury in the presence of pelvic fracture:

■ Blood at the opening of the urethral meatus
■ Scrotal or labial hematoma
■ High-riding prostate on rectal examination (Figs 4-6)

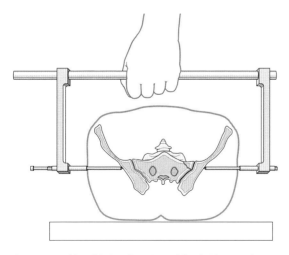

Fig 4-5 Unstable pelvic ring disruption stabilized with external pelvic resuscitation clamp.

Blind insertion of a urinary catheter may convert a partial urethral rupture into a complete one in males. If in doubt, a retrograde urethrogram should be performed before a urinary catheter is inserted.

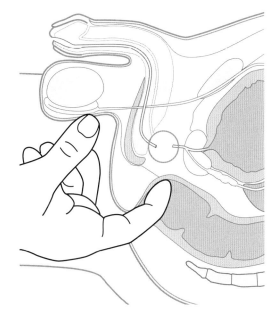

Fig 4-6 High-riding prostate due to urethral rupture on rectal examination.

4.4   Second phase (1–24 hours)

After respiratory and hemodynamic stabilization, the clinical and x-ray examinations are completed. Next the integral management of all relevant injuries follows.

Long-bone fractures

Unstable fractures of the femur, tibia, and humerus should in principle be stabilized within 24 hours to reduce blood loss, minimize pain, facilitate nursing, and in particular to prevent secondary pulmonary problems (adult respiratory distress syndrome). In the acute phase, fractures can be stabilized temporarily with external fixation. This is a concept called damage-control orthopaedics (DCO).

The estimated blood loss in closed fractures is (Fig 4-7):

- Pelvis: 1,000–4,000 mL
- Femur: 1,000–2,500 mL
- Tibia: 500–1,500 mL
- Humerus: 200–500 mL
- Radius/ulna: 280–400 mL

   ■ The blood loss in open fractures can be much larger due to the soft-tissue injury and loss of temponade.

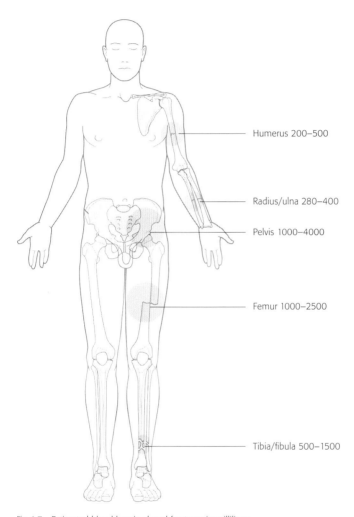

Humerus 200–500

Radius/ulna 280–400

Pelvis 1000–4000

Femur 1000–2500

Tibia/fibula 500–1500

Fig 4-7   Estimated blood loss in closed fractures in milliliters.

Open fractures

Due to increasing risk of infection as time passes, open fractures should be treated as a priority. Debridement of devitalized soft tissue is the basis of all treatment. Whether traumatic wounds are closed or left open depends on the location, soft-tissue edema, the degree of contamination, and the extent of soft-tissue damage.

- Patients with open injuries should receive tetanus prophylaxis.
- Open fractures should be treated for 24 hours with a first-generation cephalosporin to reduce risk of infection.

Patients with crush injuries are at risk for the following conditions:
- Compartment syndrome may develop in this situation and fasciotomy is frequently indicated (see chapter 14).
- Myoglobinuria—causing acute tubular necrosis; therefore, aggressive fluid resuscitation to ensure forced diuresis and alkalinization of the urine is necessary.

Injuries associated with risk of loss of limbs:
- Open fractures
- Dislocation of large joints
- Crush injuries
- Vascular injuries
- Compartment syndrome

4.5 Third phase (1–5 days)

In a stabilized patient, semielective surgery is performed. Fractures that may be repaired in this phase are intraarticular fractures and closed fractures of the short bones.

4.6 Fourth phase (from the 6th day)

Unstable vertebral fractures not associated with neurological deterioration in which surgery is indicated can be safely reduced and fixed in this phase. The same applies to ligament injuries (knee and elbow), acetabular and pelvic fractures, or calcaneal fractures.

Skull/brain injury

0	=	no injury
1	=	skull injury without loss of consciousness
2	=	loss of consciousness < 15 min, fracture of the skull, minor facial injuries, neck pain without fracture
3	=	loss of consciousness for 15–60 min, impression fracture, serious facial fractures, spinal cord fracture without neurological deficit
4	=	loss of consciousness for >60 min or focal signs, spinal cord fracture with paraplegia, unconsciousness without response >24 hours (EMV = 3)
5	=	spinal cord fracture with high paraplegia (tetraplegia)

Respiratory injury

0	=	no injury
1	=	contusion of thorax wall, no objective abnormalities
2	=	rib fracture, sternum fracture, lung contusion
3	=	fractured first rib, several fractured ribs, hemothorax, pneumothorax
4	=	open pneumothorax, tension pneumothorax, flail chest, ruptured diaphragm, ruptured trachea
5	=	aspiration, bilateral flail chest, bilateral lung contusion, tension pneumothorax with shock

Table 4-1　Injury Severity Scale (ISS) to evaluate polytrauma patients within 24 hours of admission.

Cardiovascular injury

0	=	no injury
1	=	<500 mL blood loss, normal capillary refill
2	=	500–1000 mL blood loss, reduced capillary refill, heart contusion
3	=	1000–1500 mL blood loss with blood pressure (BP) <100 mm Hg, heart contusion with drop in BP, tamponade with normal BP
4	=	1500–2000 mL blood loss with BP <80 mm Hg, tamponade with drop in BP
5	=	>2000 mL blood loss with BP <60 mm Hg, cardiac arrest due to bleeding

Abdominal injury

0	=	no injury
1	=	contusion of abdominal wall or side, without signs of peritonitis
2	=	local peritonitis of abdomen or side, fractured ribs 7–12, hematuria
3	=	ruptured liver grade 1–2, small intestine, spleen, body of pancreas, mesentery, ureter, urethra, several fractured ribs 7–12
4	=	ruptured liver grade 3–4, bladder, head of pancreas, duodenum, colon, large tear in mesentery
5	=	ruptured liver grade 5–6, great vessels (including thoracoaortic rupture), aorta, vena cava/iliac/hepatic arteries

Table 4-1   (cont) Injury Severity Scale (ISS) to evaluate polytrauma patients within 24 hours of admission.

Limbs injury

0	=	no injury
1	=	contusions and fractures, excluding long bones
2	=	humerus, clavicle, lower arm, lower leg, minor neurological deficit, simple luxation
3	=	multiple fractures or open fractures of the above, femur, stable pelvic fracture, thoracolumbar vertebrae, serious injury of the nervous system (plexus), serious displacement fracture
4	=	two of above fractures, open fracture of femur, crushed limb, traumatic amputation, unstable pelvic ring, unstable fracture thoracolumbal vertebrae
5	=	multiple injuries with score 3, two injuries with score 4, open crush injury of pelvis ring

Soft-tissue injury

0	=	no injury
1	=	<5% burns, abrasions, contusion, or wounds
2	=	5–15% burns, extensive abrasions, contusions, or wounds
3	=	15–30% burns, avulsion of soft tissues $<30 \times 30$ cm
4	=	30–45% burns, avulsion of whole limb
5	=	>45% burns

Table 4-1 (cont) Injury Severity Scale (ISS) to evaluate polytrauma patients within 24 hours of admission.

The ISS is the total of the square of the three highest scores.

Example

Skull brain injury

Loss of conciousness for >68 min or focal signs = 4

Respiratory injury

Contusion of thorax wall = 1

Cardiovascular injury

1500 mL blood loss with BP
< 100 mm Hg = 3

Abdominal injury

No injury = 0

Limbs injury

Fractured humerus = 2

Soft-tissue injury

No injury = 0

Example: 3 highest scores are squared, eg, 4, 3 and 2: 16 + 9 + 4 = 29

Table 4-1   (cont) Injury Severity Scale (ISS) to evaluate polytrauma patients within 24 hours of admission.

Part II

5 Shoulder and humerus injuries

5 Shoulder and humerus injuries

5.1 Clavicle fractures

Mechanism of injury

Direct force caused by a fall on the shoulder and upper arm; or indirect force, a fall on an outstretched arm or the elbow.

Clinical presentation

Depending on the force of the impact, there will be obvious external displacement. In children a greenstick fracture is often seen with slight swelling and tenting of the skin. In adults there is a painful swelling and the end of the bone may be prominent.

Diagnostics

Physical examination: Deformed contour, local pain on palpation; abnormal mobility in case of displacement.

X-ray examination: If the diagnosis is clear clinically, an x-ray is not always necessary. Generally, an AP view is sufficient.

Classification

- Fracture of the shaft: most fractures occur at the junction of the middle 1/3 and lateral 1/3 of the clavicle (Fig 5-1)
- Lateral fracture (Fig 5-2)
- Medial fracture

Treatment

Conservative treatment: Used for most fractures of the shaft, with a sling for 1–3 weeks, depending on pain and degree of displacement.

Surgical treatment: For fractures in the lateral part of the clavicle when there is considerable instability and displacement due to injury to the ligaments between the coracoid and clavicle or in open fractures (Figs 5-3, 5-4). Surgery is also indicated in cases of nonunion.

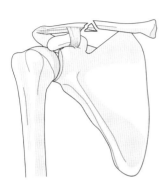

Fig 5-1   Characteristic site of a fracture of the clavicular shaft with one butterfly fragment.

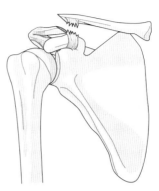

Fig 5-2   Fracture of the lateral part of the clavicle with injury to the ligaments.

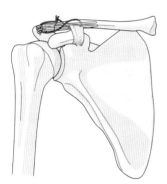

Fig 5-3   Lateral clavicular fracture treated with a tension band.

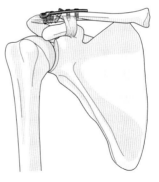

Fig 5-4   Lateral clavicular fracture treated with a plate and screws.

The surgical treatment of lateral fractures consists of a tension band, sometimes with temporary fixation across the AC joint. In comminuted fractures, plate osteosynthesis can be considered.

Surgical treatment is indicated in shaft fractures with threatened damage to the skin (rare) or neurovascular injury. Other displaced fractures may be treated surgically according to surgeon and patient preference. For osteosynthesis of shaft fractures, a plate and screws or an intramedullary pin is used. Pseudarthrosis of the clavicular shaft is also treated with plate osteosynthesis, combined with bone grafting if necessary. A tension band is used in pseudarthrosis of the lateral part of the clavicle.

Follow-up treatment: Functional with a sling for 2–4 weeks. Transarticular fixation material should be removed after 6 weeks. Until then, the arm should not be abducted more than 90°.

Duration

Fracture takes 4–8 weeks to heal.

Duration of disability is 3–8 weeks and strongly dependent on the patient's profession and the load to the shoulder girdle.

Prognosis

Prognosis is normally good. Pseudarthrosis rarely occurs. Troublesome callus formation or persistent displacement after the fracture has healed can lead to local problems that may rarely need surgical treatment.

If shortening occurs as the fracture heals, the asymmetry of the shoulder girdle is well tolerated.

5.2   Sternoclavicular dislocation

Mechanism of injury

Fall on an outstretched arm or direct force to the anterior shoulder girdle.

- Watch out for preexistent, sometimes double-sided instability.

Clinical presentation

Asymmetry of the sternoclavicular junction. There is an anteroinferior displacement of the clavicle, but dislocation can also occur posteriorly into the sternum.

Diagnostics

Physical examination: Local asymmetry, pain on palpation, and an abnormal contour at the clavicular-sternum juncture.

X-ray examination: Conventional x-rays are rarely informative; tomography or computed tomographic (CT) scan is often necessary.

Classification

- Anteroinferior or superior displacement (Fig 5-5)
- Posterior displacement (Fig 5-6)

    ■ Posterior dislocation is associated with a risk of life-threatening hemorrhage from the great retrosternal vessels, and usually occurs in high-energy trauma.

Treatment

Conservative treatment: With marginal displacement. Some asymmetry may remain but does not usually cause problems. The treatment consists of a sling for 3 weeks.

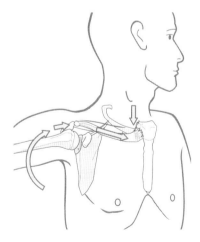

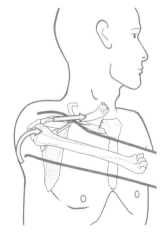

Fig 5-5   Sternoclavicular dislocation with anterior displacement.

Fig 5-6   Sternoclavicular dislocation with posterior displacement.

Surgical treatment: Only necessary for severe anteroinferior and certainly for posterior displacement. Reduction and fixation to the sternum with a plastic loop, plantaris tendon graft, or resorbable stitches. Repair of the costoclavicular ligament (the major stabilizer of the joint) is not possible.

■ Transarticular fixation with K-wires should be avoided because of the risk of wires breaking and/or migration.

Follow-up treatment: A sling and pendulum exercises of the glenohumeral joint with the arm hanging down.

Duration
Dislocation takes 3–6 weeks to heal.
Duration of disability is 2–8 weeks, depending on the subjected load.

Prognosis
Prognosis is usually good. With persistent problems such as painful crepitations and instability, a T-plasty or partial medial clavicular resection, saving the costoclavicular ligaments, may be necessary.

5.3   Acromioclavicular dislocation

Mechanism of injury
Direct injury from a fall on the shoulder associated with torsion and rolling movement.

Clinical presentation
With displacement, the patient should be examined in a standing position to emphasize the deformity of the clavicle in relation to the acromion.

Diagnostics
Physical examination: There is pain on palpation and an abnormal range of motion in the craniocaudal (piano key sign) and sometimes AP aspect.
X-ray examination: Standing AP view with arms hanging down. If in doubt take a comparative view of the nonaffected shoulder, possibly with a light weight in each hand.

Classification

Tossy classification according to the severity of the injury of the ligamentous structures:

Type I: Injury of ligaments between clavicle and acromion (distortion). No dislocation of the acromioclavicular joint (Fig 5-7).

Type II: Full tear of ligaments with a partial rupture between the coracoid process and clavicle. Restriction in range of motion in the craniocaudal direction. Partial displacement of the acromioclavicular joint (Fig 5-8).

Type III: Full rupture of ligaments between the coracoid process and clavicle. The ligaments of the inferior aspect of the clavicle can also be torn from the periosteum (often seen in young people). The clavicle is clearly displaced superiorly to the acromion; complete displacement of the acromioclavicular joint; besides craniocaudal mobility (piano key sign), there is also AP instability (Fig 5-9).

Treatment

Conservative treatment: Functional with a sling for 2–3 weeks, as pain permits.

Surgical treatment: Only used in type III injuries. The indication for surgical treatment is controversial. This is usually made for esthetic reasons and/or is dependent on the physical (sportive) activities of the patient. After reduction, the clavicle is fixed with one or two K-wires through the AC joint in combination with a strong suture around or a screw between the clavicle and coracoid process.

Follow-up treatment: Sling for 6 weeks. Transarticular fixation material should be removed after 6 weeks. Until that time, the arm should not be abducted more than 90°.

Duration

Injury takes 6–8 weeks to heal in case of a full tear, whether or not treated surgically.

Duration of disability is 2 weeks to 3 months, depending on load to the shoulder.

Prognosis

With instability the prognosis is normally good. Persistent symptoms can occur if the shoulder is under a heavy load. The indication for secondary T-plasty or resection of the distal end of the clavicle is limited.

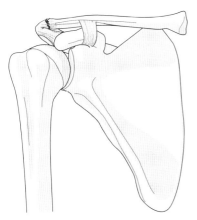

Fig 5-7   Tossy type I acromioclavicular dislocation.

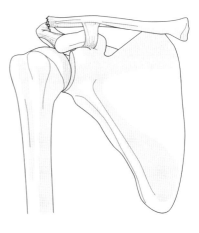

Fig 5-8   Tossy type II acromioclavicular dislocation.

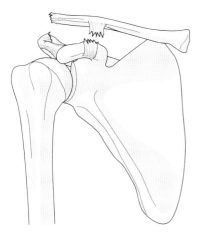

Fig 5-9   Tossy type III acromioclavicular dislocation.

5.4 Fractures of the acromion and coracoid process

Mechanism of injury
Commonly from direct force (impact to the shoulder region), and rarely occurs in a fall with an outstretched arm.

Clinical presentation
Swelling and pain to the anterosuperior aspect of the shoulder. Flexing of muscles of the upper arm is painful.

Diagnostics
Physical examination: Local pain on palpation without restricted range of motion of the clavicle.
X-ray examination: Conventional x-rays are adequate.

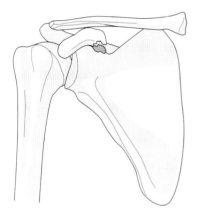

Fig 5-10   Fracture of the coracoid process.

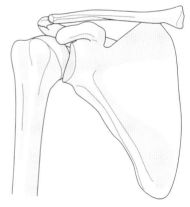

Fig 5-11   Fracture of the acromion.

Classification
None.

Treatment
Conservative treatment: For a marginally displaced fracture use a sling.
Surgical treatment: Osteosynthesis by means of cerclage or screw fixation when a major part of the acromion or coracoid is displaced, or with a combination of both.
Follow-up: Sling for 2–4 weeks and pendulum exercises with the arm hanging down.

Duration
Fracture takes 4–6 weeks to heal.
Duration of disability is also 4–6 weeks, depending on the load to the arm and shoulder.

Prognosis
Prognosis is good.

5.5   Glenoid and scapula neck fractures

Mechanism of injury
High-energy force to the lateral aspect of the upper arm with axial loading on the abducted arm.

Clinical presentation
Hematoma formation around the shoulder. Pain on all movements of the shoulder.

Diagnostics
Physical examination: Swelling and pain in the shoulder region, also in the posterior aspect if the scapula neck is fractured. All movements of the shoulder joint are painful.
X-ray examination: Conventional x-rays (including axillary views) usually give sufficient information. For optimal evaluation a CT scan is needed.

Classification
- Glenoid fracture
- Scapula neck fracture
- Combination with clavicular fracture (floating shoulder)

Treatment
Conservative treatment: For glenoid fractures if there is no or only marginal displacement; in case of severe comminuted fractures of the glenoid use sling, start exercises immediately, pendulum the arm backward and forward. In scapula neck fractures use sling and early exercises.

Surgical treatment: In fractures of the glenoid with dislocation of the humeral head. Surgical reduction and fixation is performed if the glenohumeral joint is still unstable after reduction of the dislocation. If the glenoid is split into several (often two) large fragments and with severe displacement of the scapula neck: osteosynthesis is indicated to restore the anatomical proportions as well as possible (Fig 5-12). If combined with a clavicular fracture (floating shoulder), osteosynthesis of the clavicle may be adequate (Fig 5-13).

Follow-up: Sling and start pendulum exercises immediately.

Duration
Fracture takes 6–8 weeks to heal.
Duration of disability is 2–3 months.

Prognosis
The prognosis of a glenoid fracture is good when there is no serious damage to the glenohumeral joint area. Arthrosis can occur and cause restricted shoulder function and a reduction in the load-bearing capacity of the joint when the articular surface is involved. The prognosis of a scapular fracture is good. The prognosis of a floating shoulder depends on the degree of displacement and the severity of the accompanying injury to the soft tissues.

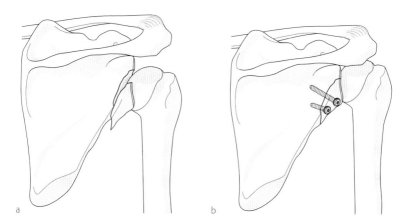

Fig 5-12a–b   Fracture of the scapula neck treated with screw osteosynthesis.

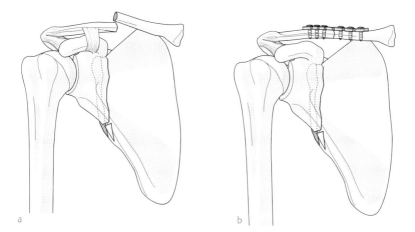

Fig 5-13a–b   Floating shoulder treated with osteosynthesis of the clavicle.

5.6   Scapula body fractures

Mechanism of injury
Usually from direct high-energy force to the shoulder blade.

Clinical presentation
Local swelling and pain, often with skin damage.

- Always consider possibility of accompanying rib fractures and/or underlying pulmonary injury.

Diagnostics
Physical examination: Local swelling and pain on palpation of the shoulder blade and a painful range of motion, mainly shoulder abduction. Pain on inspiration if a rib fracture has occurred.
X-ray examination: AP views of the shoulder, particularly the scapula (Fig 5-14).

Classification
None.

Treatment
Conservative treatment: Sling, glenohumeral and scapulothoracic movements as soon as possible; exercises may be undertaken if pain allows (swinging arm backward and forward). Strong analgesia is required for the first 48 hours.
Surgical treatment: Usually not indicated.

Duration
Fracture takes 3–4 weeks to heal.
Duration of disability is 4–6 weeks.

Prognosis
Prognosis is good.

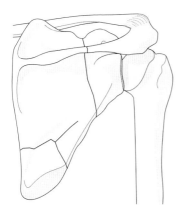

Fig 5-14 Fracture of the scapula body.

5.7 Anterior glenohumeral dislocation

Mechanism of injury

The dislocation usually occurs due to a fall on the hand and/or arm when external rotation of the shoulder occurs. The arm is usually in abduction in relation to the trunk. The injury most frequently occurs in people aged 18 to 25 years (sport or motorbike injuries) and in the elderly (falls with the arm outstretched).

Clinical presentation

As the head of the humerus is displaced anteriorly to the joint and lies anterior to the scapula neck, there is local pain and swelling. Sometimes the normal rounded contour of the shoulder is lost. The injured arm is supported by the unaffected hand and all movements are avoided (Fig 5-15).

Diagnostics

Physical examination: On careful palpation under the acromion, the humeral head is not in situ. The displaced humeral head can be felt anteriorly to the shoulder. The axis of the upper arm is more medial than on the healthy side.

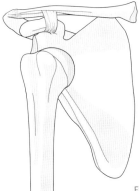

Fig 5-15   Glenohumeral dislocation with anterior displacement.

■ Look for signs of neurological deficit (axillary nerve) and injury of the axillary artery. In the acute stage, paralysis due to damage to the axillary nerve can only be shown by hypesthesia in the deltoid region, since pain prevents testing the function of the deltoid muscle.

X-ray examination: Conventional x-rays in two planes are adequate. They show an anteromedial displacement of the humeral head toward the glenoid. A fracture or avulsion of the anterior aspect of the glenoid rim (Boney Bankart lesion) may be visible, particularly on x-ray after reduction. In the elderly, an avulsion of the greater tuberosity is often seen. If in doubt, a lateral/axillary view can be useful. If the shoulder is too painful for this view, a transthoracic view is indicated.

Classification
Classification according to the site of the displacement of the humeral head with respect to the glenoid (subglenoidal, subcoracoidal, or subclavicular) is not relevant.

Treatment
Conservative treatment: Reduction of the displaced humeral head. Administer intraarticular local anesthetics. The Kocher and Hippocrates methods are often used (Fig 5-16), as well as hanging a weight from the wrist with the patient in prone position (Fig 15-17). If reduction of the joint is not achieved in this way, reduction under sedation is necessary.

■ There is a risk of humeral fracture with the Kocher method.

Surgical treatment: Open reduction is reserved for chronic dislocation or acute dislocation with a completely displaced proximal humeral fracture. If an associated greater tuberosity fragment is still displaced after reduction of the dislocation, it should be reduced and fixed at time of surgery.

Follow-up: A sling or antirotation brace for 3 weeks. Start pendulum exercises after 1 week. External rotation should be avoided for the first weeks.

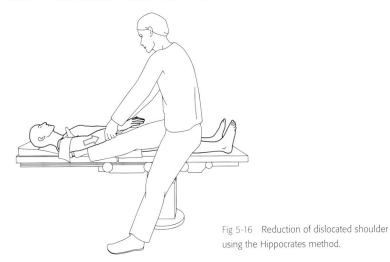

Fig 5-16   Reduction of dislocated shoulder using the Hippocrates method.

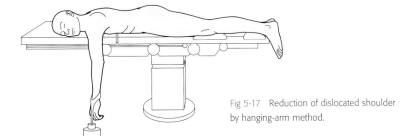

Fig 5-17   Reduction of dislocated shoulder by hanging-arm method.

Duration
Injury takes 4–6 weeks to heal.
Duration of disability is also 4–6 weeks, depending on load to the arm and shoulder.

Prognosis
Prognosis in the elderly is good.

- Be cautious of frozen shoulder.

In young patients the risk of reoccurring dislocation is considerable, mainly in case of a Bankart lesion.

5.8 Posterior glenohumeral dislocation

Mechanism of injury
Usually from a fall on an outstretched, internally rotated arm or by direct force to the anterior aspect of the shoulder. This injury can also occur during a seizure.

Clinical presentation
The shoulder is kept fixed and the contour is abnormal on both the anterior and posterior aspect of the joint. Movement is painful and avoided by the patient, mainly external rotation.

- Diagnosis is often missed.

Diagnostics
Physical examination: The normal contour of the shoulder is lost. The shoulder is held in internal rotation.

X-ray examination: X-rays are important. On AP view, posterior displacement is often missed. The humeral head appears to be "smaller" in comparison with the glenoid (Fig 5-18). On a lateral x-ray, posterior dislocation can be seen on axillary or transthoracic views (Fig 5-19). A CT scan not only shows dislocation but also an impression fracture of the humeral head which is nearly always present as well. Other examination is not needed unless there is some neurological deficit.

■ In Erbs paralysis, a posterior dislocation is often missed.

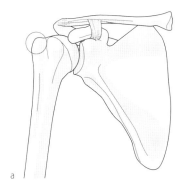
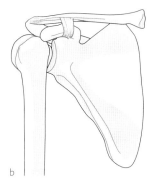

Fig 5-18a–b Glenohumoral dislocation with posterior displacement. a Normal AP view. b On AP view of posterior dislocation, the major tuberosity is not pictured. Posterior dislocation shown on axillary view.

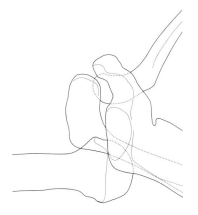

Fig 5-19 Glenohumoral dislocation with posterior displacement on axillary view on x-ray.

Classification

None.

Treatment

Conservative treatment: Traction of the arm in a position of 90° abduction with gentle external rotation.

Surgical treatment: Not indicated except for a chronic dislocation.

Follow-up treatment: With normal stability after reduction, a sling or antirotation brace. Exercises may be started early with the arm hanging, carefully preventing internal rotation, hyperabduction, and elevation. If the joint is unstable, treatment in an abduction frame or cast with the arm in 40° abduction and 60° external rotations is indicated.

Duration

Injury takes 4–6 weeks to heal.

Duration of disability is also 4–6 weeks, depending on the degree of load to the arm.

Prognosis

Prognosis is good; recurrent posterior dislocation is rare.

■ A recurrent posterior dislocation should be distinguished from the voluntary posterior dislocation that occurs with inadequate musculature.

5.9   Inferior glenohumeral dislocation (luxatio erecta)

Mechanism of injury

Forced traction of the arm with hyperabduction or displacing the humeral head inferiorly, such as a fall from a tree or gymnastic apparatus.

Clinical presentation

The arm is held vertically and is painful on all attempts to bring it into a normal position.

Diagnostics

Physical examination: A vacant space is felt under the acromion. The shoulder area is swollen, painful, and the patient avoids all movements.

X-ray examination: Conventional AP views.

Classification
None.

Treatment
Conservative treatment: Reduction with traction in abduction, with the arm in a neutral position. Use careful adduction movements.

■ Be alert for injury to the axillary nerve.

Surgical treatment: None.
Follow-up treatment: Sling or antirotation brace for 3 weeks, then exercises followed by muscle training.

Duration
Injury takes 4–6 weeks to heal.
Duration of disability is also 4–6 weeks.

Prognosis
Prognosis is good; with injury of the axillary nerve, the prognosis is uncertain.

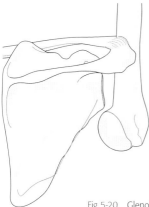

Fig 5-20   Glenohumeral dislocation with inferior displacement (luxatio erecta).

5.10   Rotator cuff injuries

Mechanism of injury
Traumatic ruptures of the rotator cuff are rare because a fracture of the greater tuberosity is more likely to occur. The supraspinatus is usually injured (Fig 5-21). The injury can occur due to extreme acute traction.

Most injuries of this type occur in older people and are of a degenerative nature. Often this degeneration is insidious and partial tears occur, which can be exacerbated by trauma resulting in total rupture.

Clinical presentation
Presenting with acute pain in the anterior aspect of the shoulder. The patient cannot actively lift or abduct the arm.

Diagnostics
Physical examination: There is pain on local palpation of the anterior aspect of the shoulder and subacromion. Abduction against resistance is painful and cannot be carried out.
X-ray examination: In a long-standing rotator cuff rupture, the humeral head lies anteriorly to the glenoid.
Supplementary examinations: Arthrography, ultrasound, and MRI can show the rupture. The size of the rupture can also be determined.

Classification
A distinction is made between complete and partial ruptures. The clinical picture can also give an impression of the site of the rupture in the supraspinatus or in the infraspinatus area.

Treatment
Conservative treatment: For ruptures caused by degeneration in older patients.
Surgical treatment: In younger patients with an acute rupture. An attempt is made to suture the rupture, if necessary also combined with an acromionplasty to increase the subacromial space. If the rupture cannot simply be sutured, an acromionplasty may be enough to relieve symptoms. Surgery is frequently performed arthroscopically.

Follow-up treatment: After suturing the rupture, immobilize for 6 weeks in a sling. The shoulder may not be actively abducted or elevated. As soon as possible start exercises involving swinging the arm backward and forward, while bending forward.

Duration
Injury takes 6–10 weeks to heal, depending on the severity of the rupture and the quality of the sutured tissue. Six weeks is sufficient for an acromionplasty. Duration of disability is 2–3 months, depending on the severity of the abnormality and the quality of the tissues.

Prognosis
Prognosis in the elderly is poor; in young patients, good.

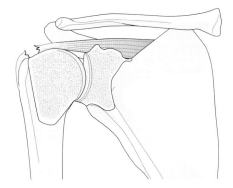

Fig 5-21   Rupture of the tendon of the supraspinatus muscle.

5.11   Labral injuries

Mechanism of injury
Dislocation of the shoulder. The site of the labral injury depends on the direction of the humeral head displacement. These injuries particularly occur in people taking part in ball sports, such as pitchers in baseball or basketball.

Clinical presentation
Presenting with symptoms in the shoulder on maximal elevation or abduction and with quick, forceful movements.

Diagnostics
Physical examination: Positive apprehension test and local pain on maximal elevation and retroflexion of the abducted arm.
X-ray examination: Conventional x-rays do not show any abnormalities. Labral injury can be demonstrated on ultrasound. The diagnosis can be confirmed by MRI or arthroscopy.

Classification
None.

Treatment
Conservative treatment: Avoid maximal loading or adapt sporting activities.
Surgical treatment: Arthroscopic or open suturing of the labrum to the edge of the glenoid.
Follow-up treatment: Antirotation braces, and start pendulum exercises immediately followed by muscle training.

Duration
Injury takes 6–8 weeks to heal.
Duration of disability is also 6–8 weeks.

Prognosis
Prognosis is usually good in surgically treated patients.

5.12   Biceps muscle rupture

Mechanism of injury
Abrupt uncoordinated flexion of the biceps muscle, eg, due to lifting a heavy object. Usually a rupture occurs in a tendon that is already showing degenerative changes in the part where the long biceps muscle enters the shoulder joint (usually the sulcus). Avulsion of the attachment point can also occur. A distal rupture of the biceps muscle at the level of the insertion of the radius is rare.

Clinical presentation
Present with painful upper arm with swelling of thickest part of the muscle that increases on flexing the muscles (Fig 5-22).

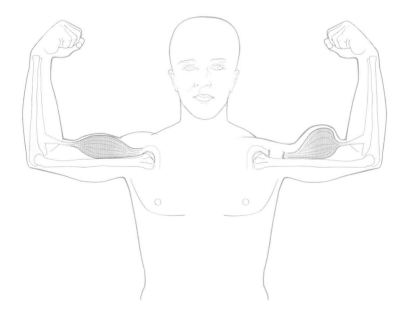

Fig 5-22   Prominent muscle bulge with a rupture of the long tendon of the biceps muscle.

Diagnostics

Physical examination: Swelling, pain, and hematoma formation at the anterior aspect of the upper arm, a clearly visible bulging contraction of the part of the muscle active in flexing the biceps muscle. In case of a rupture, active flexion of the elbow is difficult. With a distal rupture, there is a loss of strength in the flexion of the elbow and supination of the forearm.

X-ray examination: None.

Classification

None.

Treatment

Conservative treatment: Use for most degenerative tears of the long tendon. Symptomatic treatment and early active exercises.

Surgical treatment: Use in acute situations in young people or in patients in whom the contour of the torn biceps muscle is causing problems. Anatomical reconstruction should not be the goal, but rather repair of the torn tendon as proximally as possible to the humeral shaft (tenodesis). With a distal tear, reattachment to the radius is needed.

■ The surgical approach required for this repair may endanger the posterior interosseous nerve.

Follow-up treatment: 4 weeks of rest postoperatively, with exercises avoiding active flexion of the elbow.

Duration

Takes 4–6 weeks to heal.

Duration of disability is also 4–6 weeks after surgery. After conservative treatment, the degree of disability is slight and only lasts 2–3 weeks at the most.

Prognosis

Prognosis is good after both functional and surgical treatment.

5.13   Head or neck fractures of the proximal humerus

Mechanism of injury
Fall on the lateral aspect of the upper arm or on an outstretched arm.

Clinical presentation
Pain in the shoulder and upper arm; patients typically present with the injured arm supported by the other arm. There is normally little hematoma formation.

Diagnostics
Physical examination: Pain in the shoulder and upper arm region on pressure and attempts to move the arm.
X-ray examination: An x-ray in two planes shows a fracture of the head or the anatomical neck. Nondisplaced fractures are sometimes difficult to see on x-rays.

Classification
The currently used classifications (Müller AO Classification, Fig 5-23, and Neer) are not practical. To avoid a system that it is too complicated, these fractures can be classified in two groups:

- Fractures of the humeral head and through the anatomical neck (Fig 5-24)
- Fractures of the greater tuberosity

A subclassification is of little use for fractures of the head and anatomical neck. However, the degree of displacement and the number of fracture fragments is important. Müller AO Classification: 11-A1, 11-B(1–3), 11-C(1–3).

Treatment
Conservative treatment: Sling for a fracture that is not dislocated or displaced and for a head fracture with two fragments. In case of displacement, after reduction under sedation, a sling can be used for several weeks.
Surgical treatment: In older patients, a multifragmentary head fracture is primarily treated with a humeral prosthesis. Fixation of fragments by means of conventional osteosynthesis provides poor results in head fractures and anatomical neck fractures but is often the only option in young patients. Locked internal fixators provide better anchorage in osteoporotic bone and may provide stable fixation in multifragmentary fracture even in the elderly.
Follow-up treatment: Sling for several weeks, careful exercises starting with swinging the arm backward and forward as pain permits. After prosthesis, the

arm should be immobilized for 3–5 days, and then carefully mobilized with passive pendulum movements. Active mobility is allowed after 14 days.

Duration
Fracture takes 4–8 weeks to heal.
Duration of disability is 6–12 weeks.

Prognosis
Prognosis is strongly dependent on the vitality of the humeral head. The most important complication is avascular necrosis of the humeral head, although this does not necessarily lead to serious problems for the patient.

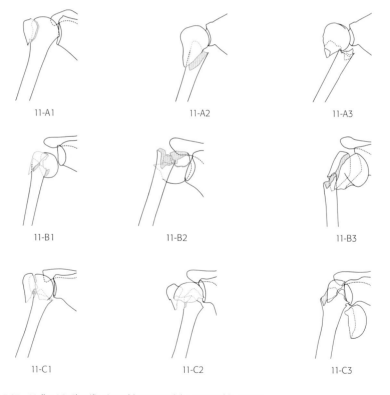

11-A1   11-A2   11-A3

11-B1   11-B2   11-B3

11-C1   11-C2   11-C3

Fig 5-23   Müller AO Classification of fractures of the proximal humerus.
This classification is complex.

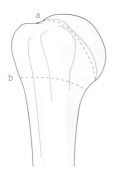

Fig 5-24   Proximal humerus: a anatomical
neck; b surgical neck.

5.14   Fractures of the humeral tuberosities

Mechanism of injury
Fall on an outstretched arm. A fracture of the greater tuberosity can occur with
shoulder dislocation (Fig 5-25). With multifragmentary fractures of the proximal
humerus, the tuberosities are usually involved.

Clinical presentation
Present with pain in the shoulder/upper arm and inability to raise the arm or
to abduct it.

■ Be alert for accompanying injury to the brachial plexus.

Diagnostics
Physical examination: Pain on palpation of the shoulder/upper arm at the
level of the greater tuberosity. The arm cannot be actively abducted. Passive
movements, chiefly rotations, are less painful.
X-ray examination: X-rays in two planes. On AP view, the greater tuberosity
is clearly visible.

Classification
According to the degree of displacement.

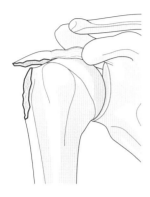

Fig 5-25   Fracture of the greater tuberosity with displacement due to traction of the supraspinatus muscle.

Treatment

Conservative treatment: If there is little or no displacement. In older patients, a slight displacement can be accepted and treated conservatively. The treatment consists of a sling for 14 days, followed by immobilization with a sling for a further 14 days. From the start, gentle passive exercises (pendulum) are possible; active abduction should not be undertaken until after 4–6 weeks, as the pain permits.

Surgical treatment: If there is displacement of the greater tuberosity (into the subacromial space). Fixation can be performed using a traction screw and/or tension band.

Follow-up treatment: Sling for 4 weeks, with pendulum exercises. Start active exercise, including abduction, only after 4–6 weeks.

Duration

Fracture takes 4–6 weeks to heal.
Duration of disability is 6–8 weeks.

Prognosis

Prognosis is good.

5.15 Surgical neck fractures of the proximal humerus

Mechanism of injury
Fall with impact on the lateral aspect of the upper arm, direct force to the upper arm, or fall on an outstretched arm. The degree of displacement and the number of fracture fragments depend on the quality of the bone and the impact of the direct force.

Clinical presentation
Pain in the upper arm at rest and increasing with movement. The hematoma can extend to the elbow and even to the hand.

Diagnostics
Physical examination: Pain in the shoulder/upper arm on palpation and with every movement. Crepitation can be heard and felt on movement.
X-ray examination: X-rays in two planes are normally adequate, but specific supplementary x-rays are sometimes necessary.

Classification
The number of fragments, degree of displacement of the fracture fragments, and of the dislocation in the head or part of the head should be considered. Of importance is whether the greater and/or lesser tuberosities are involved. Müller AO Classification: 11-A(2–3), 11-B(1–3).

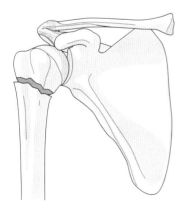

Fig 5-26   Surgical neck fracture of the proximal humerus through the surgical neck.

Treatment

Conservative treatment: If there are not many fragments and no serious displacement. With a transverse subcapital fracture, an angulation of 30° can be accepted. By using a sling to support the arm, a certain amount of reduction often occurs if angulation is present. In a nondisplaced fracture, a sling is usually used initially. Passive pendulum exercises can soon be started, depending on the pain and the degree of displacement; active movement should not be started until sufficient consolidation has been achieved after 6–8 weeks.

Surgical treatment: With multiple fragments and/or dislocation of the head or part of the head. Consider surgical fixation in three-fragment fractures when the greater and/or lesser tuberosity is fractured or displaced. Fractures with more than three fragments can be treated by osteosynthesis; in older patients with severe displacement and/or dislocation, the treatment of choice is head-neck prosthesis. The osteosynthesis should be as simple as possible because the use of large implants increases the risk of necrosis of the head. When inserting head-neck prosthesis, the greater and lesser tuberosities should be fixed around the prosthesis.

Follow-up treatment: After osteosynthesis with cerclage, pins, and/or screws, a sling should be worn for 14 days. Gentle pendulum exercises can be started after 5 days. Passive motion can then be initiated. Active exercises can begin after 5–6 weeks only after consolidation.

Duration

Fracture takes 6–8 weeks to heal.
Duration of disability is 8–10 weeks.

Prognosis

The prognosis varies considerably according to the number of fracture fragments, the vitality of the humeral head, and the damage to the soft tissues. A restriction in the range of motion often remains, chiefly of external rotation and abduction/elevation. After head-neck prosthesis, full recovery and restoration of full mobility is rarely achieved.

5.16 Injuries of the metaphysis of the proximal humerus in children

Mechanism of injury
Indirect force from a fall on an outstretched arm, direct force to the upper arm, or a blow. Birth trauma.

Clinical presentation
Pain in the upper arm at rest and increasing with movement. The child holds the arm tightly, supported by the other arm.

Diagnostics
Physical examination: Pain in the shoulder/upper arm on loading and with all movements. Local swelling.

- Be alert for accompanying injury to the brachial plexus.

X-ray examination: X-rays of the shoulder in two planes.

Classification
Metaphysis injuries can be classified according to Salter-Harris. In the proximal humerus usually only epiphysiolysis (Salter-Harris type I) and epiphysiolysis with metaphyseal fragment (Salter-Harris type II) occur.

- The epiphysis of the proximal humerus is not yet visible on x-rays in newborn infants. If in doubt, use ultrasound or MRI.

Treatment
Conservative treatment: If there is only slight displacement, in children ≤40° angulation; in adolescents ≤5°. Use Velpeau bandage or sling for 2–3 weeks. With severe displacement use closed reduction.
Surgical treatment: For severe displacement use open/closed reduction and percutaneous K-wire fixation.

- Interpositioning of the long biceps tendon or the periosteum makes closed reduction impossible in some cases. Open reduction is then indicated.

Follow-up treatment: Sling for 2–3 weeks; remove K-wires after 3 weeks.

Duration
Fracture takes 3 weeks to heal.

Prognosis
Prognosis is good. The younger a child is the greater the potential to correct angulation spontaneously.

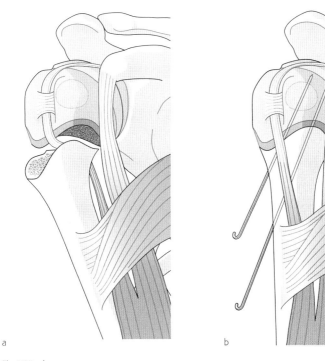

a   b

Fig 5-27a–b

a Salter-Harris type I epiphysiolysis with interposition of long head of biceps tendon.

b Same fracture treated with K-wires after open reduction.

5.17   Humeral shaft fractures

Mechanism of injury
Direct force, such as a blow or fall on the upper arm and (indirectly) through a fall on an outstretched arm. Sometimes caused by torsion force.

Clinical presentation
Swelling and pain in the upper arm; the patient supports the injured forearm with the other arm.

Diagnostics
Physical examination: Pain on palpation and on all attempts to move the arm.
X-ray examination: X-ray in two planes.

- Always check for injury to radial nerve.

Classification
Shaft fractures are classified according to location, degree of displacement, single or multiple, comminuted, and according to severity of soft-tissue injury; Müller AO Classification (Fig 5-28).

Treatment
Conservative treatment: If there is an acceptable axis and if the soft tissue is intact: coaptation splint or sling. When swelling is reduced after 1–2 weeks, this can be replaced by a functional (Sarmiento) brace.

Surgical treatment: Plates and screws or intramedullary nails are used in open fractures with serious soft-tissue injuries, bilateral fractures, and in polytrauma patients. Other indications are mainly determined by the preference of the treating surgeon or the patient. Note: Primary radial nerve paralysis is not an indication for surgery. If symptoms of radial nerve paralysis develop during conservative treatment especially after closed reduction, surgical fixation in combination with neurolysis may be indicated.

Follow-up treatment: Sling for 2 weeks, begin pendulum exercises of the shoulder, and flexion/extension exercises of the elbow as soon as possible. Start active exercises of the elbow and shoulder after 2 weeks.

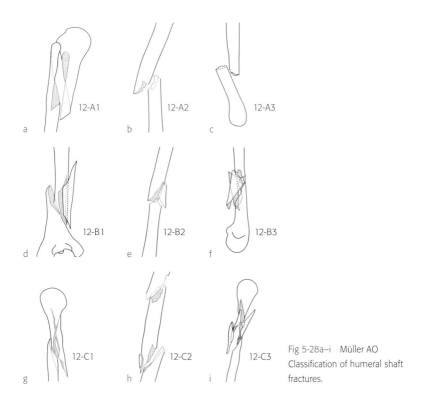

Fig 5-28a–i   Müller AO Classification of humeral shaft fractures.

Duration

Fracture takes 6–8 weeks to heal.
Duration of disability is 6–10 weeks.

Prognosis

Usually prognosis is good, also in case of paralysis of the radial nerve which resolves spontaneously in 90% of cases.

6   Elbow and forearm injuries

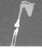

6 Elbow and forearm injuries

6.1 Supracondylar fractures of the humerus in adults

Mechanism of injury
Indirect force from a fall on an outstretched hand with hyperextension of the elbow joint. Direct force from a fall on the elbow, mainly in elderly patients with osteoporosis.

Clinical presentation
Pain in and around the elbow, swelling, obvious displacement; loss of function. The forearm looks shorter and is in pronation.

Diagnostics
Physical examination: This fracture is often associated with injuries to the skin. Local pain on palpation; active movements are also painful.

■ With severe displacement carefully assess neurovascular function, particularly to exclude compartment syndrome.

X-ray examination: X-rays of the elbow in two planes.

■ Supracondylar fractures can be associated with a proximal fracture of the humerus.

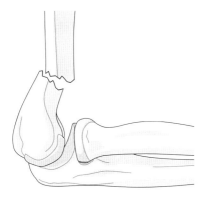

Fig 6-1 Supracondylar extension-type fracture of the humerus.

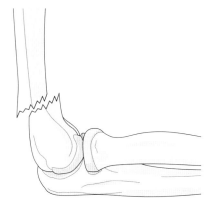

Fig 6-2 Supracondylar flexion-type fracture of the humerus is much less common.

Classification
- Extension type with dorsal displacement of the distal fracture fragment
- Flexion type with volar displacement of the distal fracture fragment
- Müller AO Classification: 13-A2, 13-A3

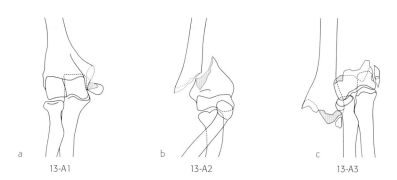

a   13-A1   b   13-A2   c   13-A3

Fig 6-3 Müller AO Classification of extraarticular fractures of the distal humerus.

Treatment

Conservative treatment: Restricted to minimally displaced fractures. These fractures generally consolidate slowly. Because of the risk of swelling under a full cast with risk of a compartment syndrome use a long arm back slab cast with the elbow flexed to 90°. When swelling is down apply a full cast for between 6–12 weeks. An alternative would be a hinged cast brace.

Surgical treatment: Open reduction and fixation of both pillars with screws, tension band, or plates with screws.

Follow-up treatment: Active exercises as soon as the wound has healed. A hinged cast brace is used postoperatively allowing flexion extension, but protecting varus valgus stresses is sometimes useful.

Duration

Fracture takes 6–8 weeks to heal.
Duration of disability is 3 months.

Prognosis

Prognosis is good; often a slight restriction in extension remains.

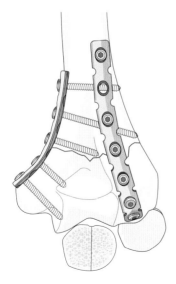

Fig 6-4   Supracondylar fracture of the humerus treated with plates and screws.

6.2 Bicondylar fractures of the humerus (T- or Y-fractures)

Mechanism of injury
Considerable direct force to the posterior aspect of the flexed elbow. This injury is most common in elderly patients with osteoporosis.

Clinical presentation
Local pain and pain with movement. Swelling, bruising, and obvious deformity.

Diagnostics
Physical examination: Tenderness on palpation, active movements are painful. Often an open fracture. Usually significant bruising and swelling.

- Perform a careful neurovascular assessment.

X-ray examination: X-rays of the elbow in two planes.

- Bicondylar fractures can be associated with proximal fracture of the humerus.

Classification
According to the displacement (rotation) and the number of fracture fragments. Müller AO Classification: 13-C(1–3) (Fig 6-5).

Treatment
Conservative treatment: In nondisplaced fractures (rare) use a long-arm cast with the elbow flexed to 90° for 6–8 weeks. In older patients with severe osteoporosis and a comminuted fracture, it is sometimes wise not to attempt surgical therapy. This is usually in patients with significant other medical comorbidities; the "bag-of-bones" concept is used with early active movements.
Surgical treatment: These fractures are unstable. With severe displacement of the joint area, surgery is generally indicated. After reconstruction of the joint area both pillars are stabilized, usually by means of plates and screws (Fig 6-6). An alternative treatment may be to consider a total elbow arthroplasty (TER) if the elbow articular surface is not reconstructable or in severe osteoporosis. Osteotomy of the olecranon enables better inspection of the joint and is commonly performed.
Follow-up treatment: Active exercises as soon as the wound has healed.

Duration

Fracture takes 6–12 weeks to heal.

Duration of disability is 3 months. However, a full range of movement is only rarely achieved.

Prognosis

Prognosis is only fair because full extension and flexion are seldom achieved. The resultant functioning disability is variable, largely dependent on patient requirement.

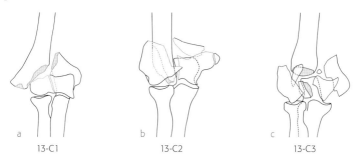

a 13-C1 b 13-C2 c 13-C3

Fig 6-5a–c Müller AO Classification of bicondylar fractures of the distal humerus.

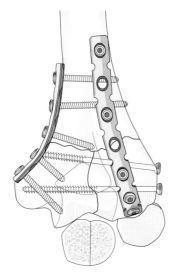

Fig 6-6 Bicondylar fracture of the humerus treated with plates and screws after lag screw fixation of the joint surface.

6.3 Supracondylar fractures of the humerus in children (extension type)

Mechanism of injury
Injury occurs due to hyperextension of the elbow with abduction or adduction caused by a fall on an outstretched arm.

Clinical presentation
Mainly in boys up to 10 years old. Pain, abnormal position of the arm, and swelling which may be gross.

Diagnostics
Physical examination: S-shaped position of the arm; generally the forearm shows internal rotation with relation to the upper arm. Local swelling (often severe) and loss of function.

- Perform a careful neurovascular assessment. Need to exclude a compartment syndrome.

X-ray examination: X-rays of the elbow in two planes. Lateral view: The ossification center of the capitulum is displaced posteriorly in relation to the humeral shaft (Fig 6-9). This short fracture line runs obliquely. In fractures with no or minimal displacement, the presence of lipo-hemarthrosis with its characteristic fat pad sign (on lateral projection) can be helpful in making the diagnosis (Fig 6-7). If in doubt, take comparative x-rays of the contralateral limb.

- Due to overprojection of fracture fragments, the x-ray is sometimes difficult to interpret.

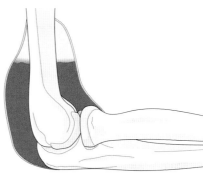

Fig 6-7 Fat pad sign with lipo-hemarthrosis of the elbow joint.

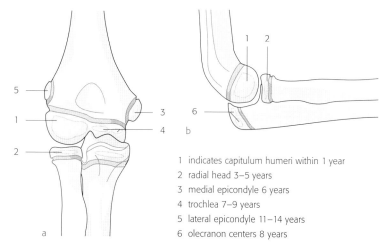

1 indicates capitulum humeri within 1 year
2 radial head 3–5 years
3 medial epicondyle 6 years
4 trochlea 7–9 years
5 lateral epicondyle 11–14 years
6 olecranon centers 8 years

Fig 6-8a–b   Ossification centers as they become visible on AP and lateral x-rays in children.

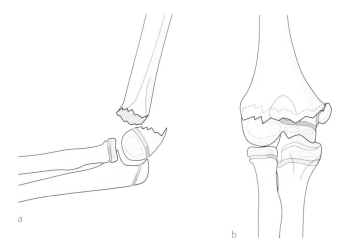

Fig 6-9a–b   Extension type of supracondylar fracture of the humerus in a child.

Treatment

Conservative treatment: In fractures with no or minimal displacement and slight swelling use a long-arm cast initially with a back slab with the elbow flexed at 90° for 3 weeks. With a displaced fracture: overhead traction for 2 weeks, then a long-arm cast for 2–3 weeks (Fig 6-10).

Surgical treatment: In most displaced fractures: closed or open reduction and fixation with K-wires (Fig 6-11), which allows postioning of elbow in any position, ie, extension if necessary. Reduction of a completely displaced fracture should be performed immediately. If swelling is great the use of overhead traction is indicated. Or nurse with the elbow extended until swelling relieved; use ice and elevation.

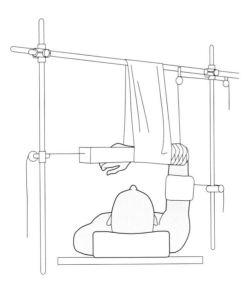

Fig 6-10   A supracondylar fracture in a child treated with overhead traction.

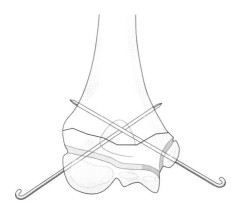

Fig 6-11 Supracondylar fracture of the humerus treated with percutaneous K-wires.

Follow-up treatment: Long-arm cast for 3 weeks, then remove K-wires.

■ Be alert for neurological injuries, vascular injuries, compartment syndrome, and Volkmann contracture.

Duration
Fracture takes 3–6 weeks to heal.

Prognosis
After anatomical reduction, a complete recovery can be expected. After nonanatomical reduction, abnormal angulation of the elbow, and restriction in extension or flexion can occur.

6.4 Supracondylar fractures of the humerus in children (flexion type)

Mechanism of injury
A fall or a blow to the flexed elbow.

Clinical presentation
The contour of the olecranon is not clearly visible. The elbow is usually held in a flexed position—a rare injury.

Diagnostics
Physical examination: Swelling of the elbow, pain, and loss of function. Needs a thorough neurovascular examination.

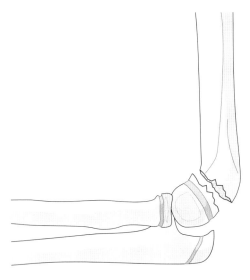

Fig 6-12   Flexion type of supracondylar fracture of the humerus in a child.

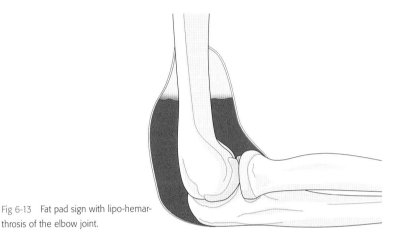

Fig 6-13   Fat pad sign with lipo-hemarthrosis of the elbow joint.

X-ray examination: X-rays of the elbow in two planes. On the lateral view, the fracture line runs in the opposite direction compared with the extension type (from anterior/proximal to dorsal/distal) (Fig 6-12). The presence of a lipo-hemarthrosis with the characteristic fat pad sign can be useful in making the diagnosis (Fig 6-13).

- Check for neurological damage, particularly to the ulnar nerve.

Treatment
Conservative treatment: In fractures with no or minimal displacement use a long-arm cast initially, and a back slab with the elbow flexed at 80–90° for 3 weeks.
Surgical treatment: In displaced fractures use closed or open reduction and fixation with K-wires.
Follow-up treatment: Long-arm cast for 3 weeks, then remove K-wires.

Duration
Fracture takes 3–6 weeks to heal depending on a patient's age.

Prognosis
After anatomical reduction a complete recovery may be expected.

6.5   Lateral condylar fractures in children

Mechanism of injury
Indirect trauma caused by a fall on an outstretched arm and supinated forearm or by a blow to the palm of the hand with the elbow flexed.

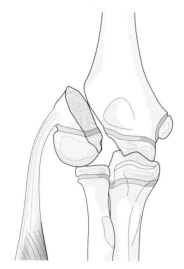

Fig 6-14   Lateral condylar fracture in a child.

Clinical presentation
Few clear symptoms, slight pain; this fracture can be missed.

Diagnostics
Physical examination: Slight swelling (hemarthrosis), pain on palpation. Range of motion, both active and passive, is not always seriously restricted.
X-ray examination: X-rays of the elbow in two planes. On AP views, a marginally displaced fracture can best be identified by a disturbed relationship between the proximal ulna and distal humerus (Fig 6-14). If a clinical diagnosis is made but x-rays fail to show an obvious fracture, take an x-ray of the normal side for comparison. Failure to diagnose this fracture may result in significant growth problems.

■ This is an injury of the epiphysis, Salter-Harris type IV.

Classification
None.

Treatment
Conservative treatment: For displacement less than 2 mm use a long-arm cast with the forearm in pronation and the elbow flexed to at least 90° for 3 weeks. Be vigilant if treating conservatively, have low threshold for K-wire treatment. X-ray after 1 week to exclude secondary displacement.

Surgical treatment: For displaced fractures use open reduction and fixation with K-wires. Accurate reduction of both growth plate and joint surface is imperative (Fig 6-15).

Follow-up treatment: Long-arm cast with the elbow flexed to 90° for 3 weeks; remove K-wires after about 6 weeks. Be careful of swelling.

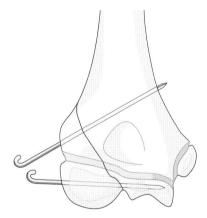

Fig 6-15   Lateral condylar fracture in a child treated with K-wires.

Duration
Fracture takes 3–6 weeks to heal.

Prognosis
The prognosis is poor if consolidation is not achieved in the anatomical position. This is caused by disruption of growth plate resulting in valgus malalignment and possible tardy ulnar nerve palsy. Also potential arthritic sequellae caused by joint surface disruption.

6.6   Medial condylar fractures in adults

Mechanism of injury
Indirect trauma caused by a fall on an outstretched hand with valgus strain on the elbow.

Clinical presentation
Pain in the elbow and restriction in range of motion. This injury rarely occurs in adults.

Diagnostics
Physical examination: Swelling, mainly at the medial aspect of the elbow. Abduction and adduction of the forearm are painful; there is restriction in the range of motion.

■ Be alert for injury of the ulnar nerve.

X-ray examination: X-rays of the elbow in two planes. The fracture is visible on the AP view; the lateral view shows little deformity.

Classification
Müller AO Classification: 13-B2.

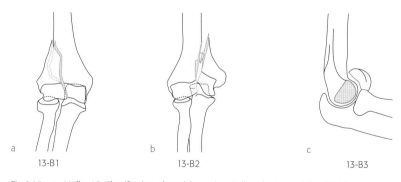

a   13-B1   b   13-B2   c   13-B3

Fig 6-16a–c   Müller AO Classification of condylar and capitellum fractures of the distal humerus, type B.

Treatment

Conservative treatment: Conservative treatment is not indicated because accurate reduction of the joint surface is required.

Surgical treatment: Screw fixation or tension band after open reduction (the ulnar nerve must be identified and protected throughout the surgical procedure). Consider anterior transposition of ulnar nerve.

Follow-up treatment: After stable fixation, initially in a hinged elbow brace, start exercises as soon as possible.

Duration

Fracture takes 6 weeks to 3 months to heal.

Duration of disability is 3 months. However, a full range of movement may not be achieved within 1 year.

Prognosis

Despite anatomical reduction and early exercises, a restriction in the range of motion often remains (loss of extension).

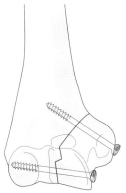

Fig 6-17   Medial condylar fracture treated with screws.

6.7   Medial condylar fractures in children

Mechanism of injury
Direct high-energy force from a fall on a flexed elbow or indirect force from a fall on an outstretched hand.

Clinical presentation
Pain in the elbow, restricted range of motion. This injury rarely occurs in children.

Diagnostics
Physical examination: Slight swelling (lipo-hemarthrosis), pain on palpation. The range of motion, both active and passive, is not always restricted. Careful examination of neurovascular status, particularly the ulnar nerve.
X-ray examination: X-rays of the elbow in two planes. Compare with the other elbow.

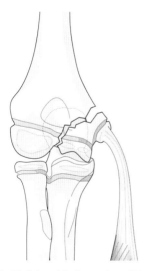

Fig 6-18   Medial condylar fracture in a child.

Classification
None.

■ Not to be confused with epicondylar fractures (see Fig 6-20).

Treatment
Conservative treatment: In nondisplaced fractures use a long-arm cast with the elbow flexed to 90° and the forearm in pronation for 3 weeks.
Surgical treatment: In displaced fractures use open reduction and K-wires (Fig 6-19).
Follow-up treatment: Long-arm cast back slab with the elbow flexed to 90° for 3 weeks; remove K-wires after about 6 weeks.

■ If the fracture is not recognized, pseudarthrosis and/or growth arrest can occur; however, this is not necessarily associated with restriction of flexion and/or extension.

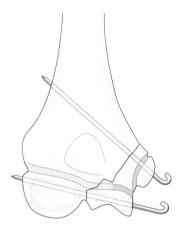

Fig 6-19   Medial condylar fracture in a child treated with K-wires.

Duration
Fracture takes 6–8 weeks to heal.

Prognosis
Prognosis is good as long as reduction is adequate.

6.8   Medial epicondyle fractures in children

Mechanism of injury
Indirect trauma from a fall on an outstretched hand with the elbow extended, so that valgus strain occurs—usually an avulsion injury of the common flexor origin.

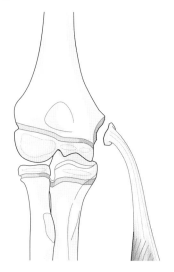

Fig 6-20   Medial epicondyle fracture in a child.

Clinical presentation
Pain and swelling, mainly at the medial aspect of the elbow; often associated with dislocation of the elbow.

Diagnostics
Physical examination: Deformity, loss of function, pain on palpation of the medial aspect.
X-ray examination: X-rays of the elbow in two planes.

- Accompanying injuries to the radial neck/head are easily missed. If there is a high suspicion of radial head injury, perform a CT scan (Fig 6-21).

- Be alert for accompanying neurological damage—ulnar nerve.

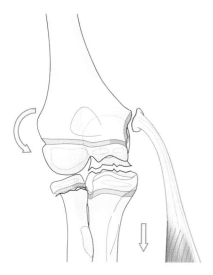

Fig 6-21   Medial epicondylar fracture with accompanying injury to the radial neck and olecranon fracture in a child.

Classification
None.

Treatment
Conservative treatment: In minimally displaced fractures use a long-arm cast with the elbow flexed to 90° and the forearm in pronation for 3 weeks.

Surgical treatment: In cases of severe displacement open reduction and K-wire fixation (Fig 6-22). Percutaneous K-wire fixation should be avoided because of the proximity of the ulna nerve.

Follow-up treatment: Long-arm cast with elbow flexed to 90° and the forearm in pronation for 3 weeks; remove K-wires about 6 weeks postoperatively.

Duration
The fracture takes 3–6 weeks to heal depending on the child's age.

Prognosis
Depending on a child's age and the degree of displacement, the prognosis after surgical treatment is good.

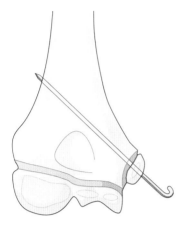

Fig 6-22   Medial epicondylar fracture in a child treated with K-wires.

6.9   Capitellum fractures (capitulum humeri)

Mechanism of injury
Indirect force from a fall on an outstretched arm: the capitellum is pushed away by the radial head.

Clinical presentation
Pain in the elbow. This injury includes the volar joint area of the lateral condyle and it is rare in children.

Diagnostics
Physical examination: The swelling is not necessarily severe, flexion is restricted.
X-ray examination: X-rays of the elbow in two planes. The fracture is usually only noticeable in the lateral view (Fig 6-23).

- Injury can be associated with fractures of the radial neck or head.

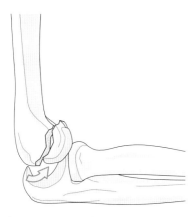

Fig 6-23 Fracture of the capitulum humeri.

Classification

- ▪ A small fragment of the capitellum
- ▪ Fracture through the major part of the lateral condyle
- ▪ Müller AO Classification: 13-B3

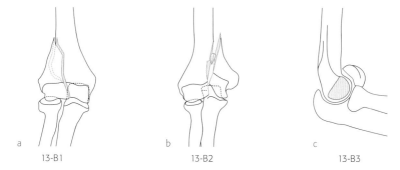

a 13-B1   b 13-B2   c 13-B3

Fig 6-24a–c Müller AO Classification of distal humerus fractures, type B (condylar and capitellum fractures).

Treatment

Conservative treatment: None.

Surgical treatment: If a small fragment is present, it is sometimes technically not possible to fix the piece of bone; the fragment is removed. With large bone fragments, treatment consists of open reduction and fixation with screws inserted dorsally (Fig 6-25). Alternatively use biodegradable screws or threaded K-wires.

Follow-up treatment: Early active exercises as soon as the wound has healed.

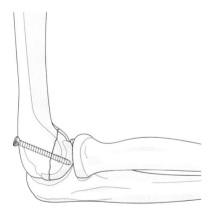

Fig 6-25   Capitellum fracture treated with a screw.

Duration

Fracture takes 2–3 months to heal.
Duration of disability is 3 months.

Prognosis

Prognosis is generally good with some restriction in range of motion (flexion and extension). Sometimes avascular necrosis of the fragment occurs with arthrosis as a result.

6.10 Olecranon fractures

Mechanism of injury
Direct force caused by a fall or blow to the posterior aspect of the elbow.
Indirect force caused by a fall on an outstretched arm or by an abrupt contraction
of the triceps muscle of the arm.

Clinical presentation
This fracture may be associated with open wounds. There is also swelling of
the elbow, pain, and the inability to actively extend the elbow.

Diagnostics
Physical examination: Swelling, local pain on palpation, and the inability to
actively extend the elbow. This can be tested against gravity.
X-ray examination: X-rays of the elbow in two planes.

Classification
Transverse, oblique, and comminuted fractures of the olecranon with or
without elbow dislocation are described (Figs 6-26, 6-27).

- Be alert for accompanying injury/dislocation of the radial head.

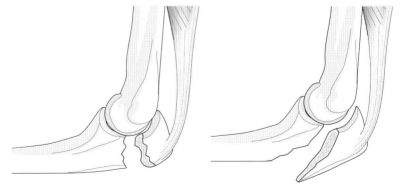

Fig 6-26   Transverse fracture of the olecranon.   Fig 6-27   Oblique fracture of the olecranon.

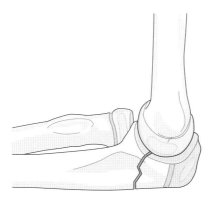

Fig 6-28 Olecranon fracture with intact extensor mechanism in a child.

In children, besides flexion-type injuries, extension injuries also occur due to an anterior hyperextension with impaction of the bone cortex on the dorsal aspect of the olecranon. The extensor mechanism is intact. This injury is rare (Fig 6-28).

Treatment

Conservative treatment: With an intact extensor mechanism, particularly in children use immobilization in a long-arm cast with the elbow flexed to 45° for 2–3 weeks.

Surgical treatment: In case of damage to the extensor mechanism use osteosynthesis by means of a tension band (Fig 6-29). In oblique fractures: screw fixation in combination with a tension band. In comminuted fractures: osteosynthesis with plate and screws (Fig 6-30).

■ In fractures of the proximal ulna including the olecranon, there is a risk of dislocation of the radial head. In such cases, this is in fact a Monteggia fracture. Check position of the radial head before and after osteosynthesis.

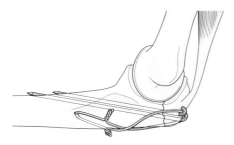

Fig 6-29 Transverse olecranon fracture treated with K-wires and tension band wiring.

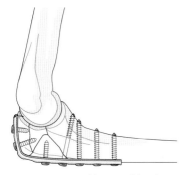

Fig 6-30 Comminuted fracture of the olecranon treated with plate and screws.

Follow-up treatment: Early active exercises to restore range of motion.

Duration
Fracture takes 6–12 weeks to heal.
Duration of disability is 6 weeks.

Prognosis
The prognosis is good. Because the material used for tension band fixation is subcutaneous, it frequently irritates the overlying skin and often needs to be removed.

6.11 Radial head fractures

Mechanism of injury
Indirect force to the shaft of the radius, such as a fall on an outstretched arm.

Clinical presentation
Swelling and pain in the lateral aspect of the elbow.

Diagnostics
Physical examination: Pain on palpation of the radial head, slight swelling of the elbow. The pain increases on supination/pronation.
X-ray examination: X-rays of the elbow in two planes. Oblique views are sometimes necessary.

- The forearm and wrist should also be examined because tearing of the interosseous membrane can occur with this injury.

- Fractures of the radial head can be associated with injuries of other anatomical structures, such as rupture of the ulnar collateral ligaments, olecranon fracture, or elbow dislocation.

Classification
Many different classifications are used, such as the Mason classification:
Type I   Marginal fracture of the radial head without displacement
Type II   Chisel fracture (Meissel fracture) in which the major part of the radial head is broken and the fracture line runs longitudinally
Type III   Comminuted fracture (crush injury)
Type IV   Associated with elbow dislocation

Treatment
Conservative treatment: In nondisplaced fractures, with joint aspiration for hemarthrosis if necessary and injection of local anesthetic. Short immobilization for 7–10 days, then exercises. The same applies for a comminuted fracture in selected cases.

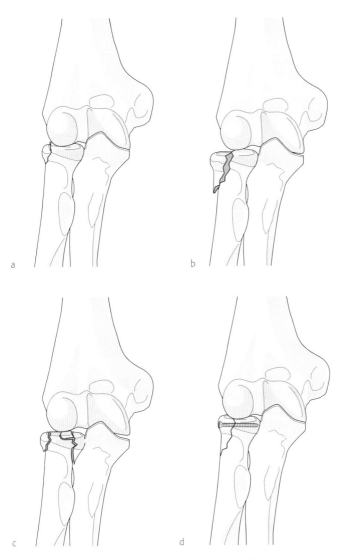

Fig 6-31a–d Fractures of the radial head. a Indicates marginal fracture, no displacement;
b chisel fracture; c comminuted fracture; and d chisel fracture of the radial head treated with
a lag screw.

Surgical treatment: In a chisel fracture with displacement of a large (>1/3) fragment use screw fixation (Fig 6-31). In a comminuted fracture: resection of the radial head combined with prosthesis if necessary (Fig 6-32). In case of accompanying injury to the ulnar collateral ligament, the aim should be to maintain the radial head, otherwise insert prosthesis.

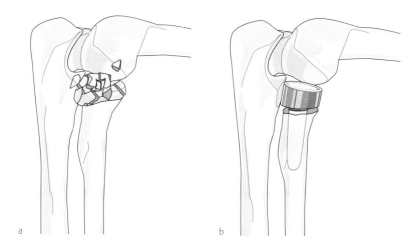

a   b

Fig 6-32a–b   Comminuted fracture of the radial head treated by resection and prosthesis.

Duration
Fracture takes 6 weeks to heal.
Duration of disability is 6 weeks to 3 months.

Prognosis
Prognosis is determined by the severity of the injury and accompanying injuries. Often restriction in rotation and extension remains. Instability is associated with a risk of arthrosis.

6.12   Radial neck fractures

Mechanism of injury
Indirect force caused by a fall on an outstretched arm.

Clinical presentation
Local pain and swelling of the joint. This injury usually occurs in children.

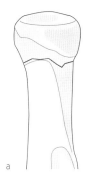

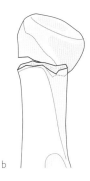

Fig 6-33a–b
a   Fracture of the radial neck without displacement.
b   Fracture of the radial neck with displacement.

Diagnostics
Physical examination: Swelling of the joint because of hemarthrosis, pain on palpation at the level of the radial head.

- Fractures of the radial neck can be associated with other injuries, such as olecranon fracture, avulsion of the medial epicondyle, and elbow dislocation.

X-ray examination: X-rays of the elbow in two planes. The fracture is most clearly seen on the AP view.

Classification
Fractures of the radial neck in children are nearly always injuries of the epiphysis (Salter-Harris type I or II). Classification is according to the degree of displacement (Fig 6-34).

Treatment

Conservative treatment: Reduction depending on the degree of displacement and the patient's age. In a child younger than 5 years a deformity of 50° is acceptable; in a child aged 5–10 years up to 30° is acceptable (Fig 6-34). Use a long-arm cast with the elbow flexed to 90° for 3 weeks.

Surgical treatment: If conservative treatment fails, such as with interposition of the annular ligament use open reduction and fixation with a K-wire or screw. Open reduction and internal fixation are also indicated when a displaced fracture occurs in an adult.

Follow-up treatment: Long-arm cast with the arm flexed to 90° for 3 weeks or functional treatment.

- Be alert for avascular necrosis of the proximal fragment.

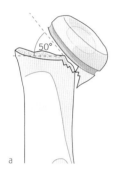 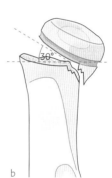

a   b

Fig 6-34a–b   Fracture of the radial neck (Salter-Harris type II). a In a child younger than 5 years, a deformity of 50° is acceptable; b in a child aged 5–10 years up to 30° is acceptable.

Duration

Fracture takes 3–4 weeks to heal in children.

Prognosis

Prognosis depends on the degree of displacement, age, accompanying injuries, and the severity of damage to soft tissues. With persistent severe displacement and avascular necrosis, prognosis is poor.

6.13 Elbow dislocations

Mechanism of injury
Indirect force from a fall on an outstretched arm together with rotation of the humeral head.

Clinical presentation
Deformity, swelling of elbow.

Diagnostics
Physical examination: Swelling, the equal-sided triangle of Hueter formed by the (epi)condyles and the top of the olecranon is no longer present (Fig 6-35); abnormal immobility, springy elastic resistance.

■ Be alert for altered sensation (neurological deficit) and absent arterial pulses (vascular injury).

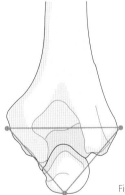

Fig 6-35   Triangle of Hueter.

X-ray examination: X-rays of the elbow in two planes. The congruity of the joint gap is disturbed. Of particular importance is the position of the radial head on the AP view.

■ Check for additional skeletal injuries, such as avulsion fractures of the medial epicondyle (about 50% of cases in children), coronoid process, radial head, or radial neck.

Classification

Dorsoradial, pure radial, or ulnar displacement; anterior dislocation or the divergent type is rare (Figs 6-36, 6-37, and 6-38).

Treatment

Conservative treatment: Closed reduction. After reduction, perform an x-ray check, assess for neurological deficit, and check arterial pulses. Always check the elbow for valgus/varus instability following reduction and if present treat in a hinged elbow brace.

Surgical treatment: When soft tissues or bone fragments are interposed (irreducible dislocation) or in case of instability.

Follow-up treatment: Immobilization with a long-arm cast with the elbow flexed to 90° for 2–3 weeks. When swelling subsides, start active exercises.

Duration

Injury takes 3–6 weeks to heal.
Duration of disability is 4–8 weeks. However, stiffness persists for several months.

Prognosis

Prognosis is generally good, with slight restriction in extension being the "biggest" problem. Prognosis is mainly determined by accompanying injuries. Ectopic bone formation sometimes occurs.

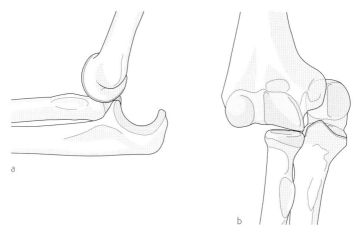

a

b

Fig 6-36a–b   Posterior dislocation of the elbow.

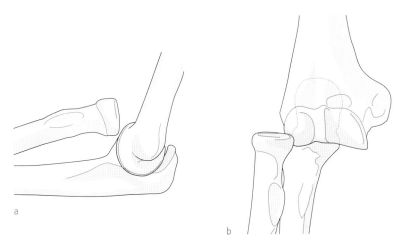

a

b

Fig 6-37a–b   Dislocation of the elbow, radial displacement.

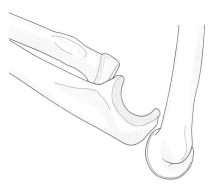

Fig 6-38   Dislocation of the elbow, anterior displacement.

6.14   Pulled elbow

Mechanism of injury

By sudden traction to an outstretched arm in children (aged 2–6 years), the annular ligament tears and part of it slides upward over the radial head.

Clinical presentation

The child does not want to use the hand and complains of pain.

Diagnostics

Physical examination: Pronation of the forearm, pain on palpation at the level of the radial head.

X-ray examination: It is debatable whether an x-ray should be taken because the case history and physical examination are usually adequate. There is controversy regarding the visibility of dislocation of the proximal radius on an x-ray.

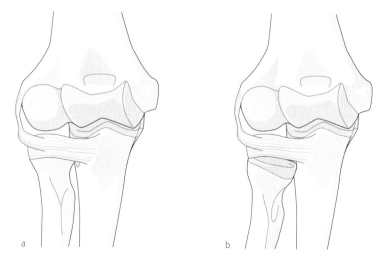

Fig 6-39a–b   Dislocation of the radial head, partly from the annular ligament. a normal anatomy; b dislocated. .

Classification

None.

Treatment

Conservative treatment: Apply pressure over the radial head, supinate and pronate the elbow as it is flexed and extended while distracting the child; a click indicates that reduction has been achieved and pain disappears straight away (Fig 6-40).
Surgical treatment: None.
Follow-up treatment: None.
Prevention: Explain the injury mechanism to the parents/caregivers.

Duration

Not applicable.

Prognosis

Prognosis is good.

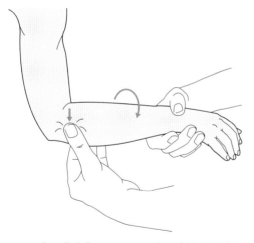

Fig 6-40 Treatment of a pulled elbow: pressure to the radial head with supination of the forearm.

6.15   Ulnar shaft fractures (proximal half) with dislocation of radial head (Monteggia fracture)

Mechanism of injury
Indirect force caused by forced pronation of the forearm or direct force, such as a fall or blow, against the dorsal aspect of the ulna.

Clinical presentation
Pain, deformity of the arm.

Diagnostics
Physical examination: Shortening of the forearm, abnormal position of the radial head, inability to move the elbow.
X-ray examination: The fracture can be seen on x-rays in two planes of the whole forearm including both wrist and elbow joints, with separate x-rays of the elbow. Radial head dislocation is often missed, chiefly in children. Thus with shortening or angulation of the ulna, attention should always be given to the correct position of the radial head and the proximal radial epiphysis in relation to the capitulum of the humerus.

■ A greenstick fracture of the ulna can be present in children with the result that radial head dislocation is not considered. Hence, always take x-rays of the elbow in angulated greenstick fractures of the ulna.

■ Check for damage to the motor branch of the radial nerve.

Classification
According to the classification of Bado, four types are distinguished:
Type I   Ulna fracture with anterior radial head dislocation (volar), the classic Monteggia fracture (Fig 6-41)
Type II   Type I with posterior dislocation (dorsal) (Fig 6-42)
Type III   Type I with lateral dislocation (particularly in children) (Fig 6-43a)
Type IV   Radial head dislocation with fractures of both radial and ulnar shaft (Fig 6-43b)

Treatment
Conservative treatment: Sometimes used in children if after reduction of the ulna, the radial head falls spontaneously into place and does not displace again. In (greenstick) fractures of the ulna use a long-arm cast for 6 weeks with the elbow flexed to 90°. On reduction of a greenstick fracture the ulna should be completely "broken" to prevent redisplacement.

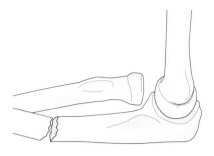

Fig 6-41 Monteggia fracture, Bado type I: ulnar fracture with anterior dislocation of the radial head.

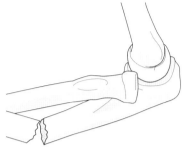

Fig 6-42 Monteggia fracture, Bado type II: ulnar fracture with dorsal dislocation of the radial head.

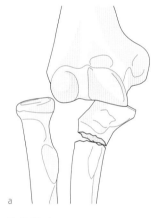

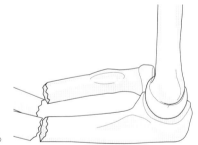

a   b

Fig 6-43a–b

a Monteggia fracture, Bado type III: ulnar fracture with radial dislocation of the radial head.

b Monteggia fracture, Bado type IV: fracture of the ulna and radius with dislocation of the radial head.

Surgical treatment: Used in all other cases. After reduction and stabilization of the ulna, the radial head nearly always returns to its anatomical position.
Follow-up treatment: Exercises as soon as the wound has healed. With conservative treatment: immobilize until consolidation of the ulna has occurred.

Duration
Fracture takes 6–12 weeks to heal.
Duration of disability is also 6–12 weeks.

Prognosis
Prognosis is good.

6.16   Radial and/or ulnar shaft fractures in adults

Mechanism of injury
Direct force to the forearm caused by a fall, blow, or impact.

Clinical presentation
Pain, deformity.

Diagnostics
Physical examination: Swelling, deformity, loss of function.
X-ray examination: X-rays in two planes of the whole of the forearm, also including wrist and elbow joints.

Classification
Shaft fractures are classified according to localization, degree of displacement, single or multiple and comminuted, open or closed, and according to the severity of soft-tissue injuries.
Müller AO Classification of forearm shaft fractures (Fig 6-44).

Treatment
Conservative treatment: In stable and only slightly displaced fractures use a long-arm cast with the elbow flexed to 90° for 8–10 weeks.
Surgical treatment: Open reduction and plate fixation. Rigid fixation is needed because of the risk of pseudarthrosis and/or synostosis (Fig 6-45).

Duration
Fracture takes 6–12 weeks to heal.
Duration of disability is 12 weeks.

Prognosis

Prognosis is good, provided an excellent reduction is obtained.

- Check for accompanying neurological damage (motor branch of the radial nerve).

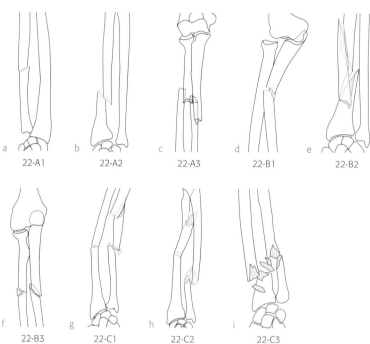

Fig 6-44a–i   Müller AO Classification of forearm shaft fractures.

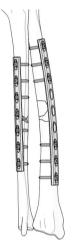

Fig 6-45   Fractures of ulnar and radial shaft treated with plates and screws.

6.17   Radial and/or ulnar shaft fractures in children

Mechanism of injury
Direct force to the forearm from a fall or blow.

Clinical presentation
Pain, deformity. These fractures often occur in children.

Diagnostics
Physical examination: Shortening of the forearm, volar angulation and radial deviation; local pain on palpation.
X-ray examination: X-rays in two planes of the whole forearm to include elbow and wrist joints.

Classification
Shaft fractures are classified according to localization, degree of displacement, fracture anatomy (simple or comminuted), open or closed, and according to the severity of soft-tissue injuries. In children incomplete and greenstick fractures often occur (Fig 6-46).

Treatment

Conservative treatment: Reduction can be done in different ways, such as by abduction of the arm, 90° flexion of the elbow, and longitudinal traction of the forearm (Fig 6-47). The result of the reduction is usually checked using an image intensifier. In a proximal fracture: long-arm cast with the elbow flexed to 90° and the forearm in pronation. In a distal fracture: the forearm in supination. If the immobilization is too short, the risk of refracture increases. Guidelines for immobilization:

- Children up to 4 years: 4 weeks
- For each additional year: 1 week longer
- If the radius and ulna are fractured at the same level: 2 weeks more
- Maximum 10 weeks

- Repeat x-rays to exclude redisplacement.

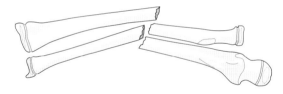

Fig 6-46   Displaced fracture of the radial and ulnar shaft in a child.

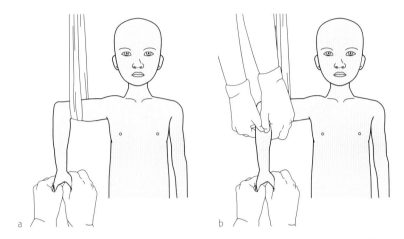

Fig 6-47a–b   Reduction of a shaft fracture of the forearm of a child by traction and manipulation.

Surgical treatment: With rotational abnormalities, interposition of soft tissues, and open fractures use open reduction and plate fixation or intramedullary osteosynthesis.

■ The degree of spontaneous positional correction depends on a patient's age, distance of the fracture from the epiphysis, degree of displacement, and direction of the angulation. From the age of 10 years onward, little spontaneous correction occurs. An axial displacement of more than 10° will hinder pronation and supination and is not acceptable.

Follow-up treatment: Functional treatment or in a long-arm cast with the elbow flexed to 90° for 4–6 weeks.

Duration
Fracture takes 4–6 weeks to heal, depending on a patient's age.

Prognosis
Prognosis is good.

■ Refracture is possible.

6.18 Radial shaft fractures with dislocation of distal radioulnar joint (Galeazzi fracture)

Fractures of the distal part of the radial shaft with dislocation of the distal radioulnar joint.

Mechanism of injury
Direct force from a fall, blow, or impact to the dorsolateral aspect of the wrist.

Clinical presentation
Pain, swelling, deformity.

Diagnostics
Physical examination: Symptoms are associated with the severity of the displacement of the radius. The distal ulna extremity may be prominent with pain on pressure to the distal radioulnar joint and pressure at the level of the fracture, compression pain.

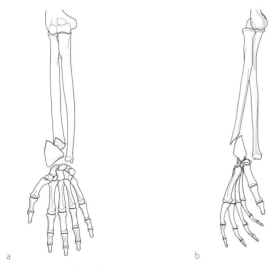

a   b

Fig 6-48a–b   Galeazzi fracture.

X-ray examination: X-rays in two planes of the whole of the forearm to include elbow and wrist joints. Also perform a separate x-ray, concentrated on the wrist, to establish incongruity of the distal radioulnar joint.

> ■ In what seems to be an isolated displaced fracture of the radial shaft, damage to the distal radioulnar joint can also be present.

Classification
Fractures classified according to Müller AO Classification (see Fig 6-44).

Treatment
Conservative treatment: None.
Surgical treatment: Open reduction and fixation of the radius to correct dislocation or subluxation of the distal radioulnar joint.
Follow-up treatment: Active exercises as soon as the wound has healed.

Duration
Fracture takes 6–12 weeks to heal.
Duration of disability is 3 months.

Prognosis
Prognosis is generally good and is mainly determined by the damage to the distal radioulnar joint.

6.19   Greenstick fractures of radial and/or ulnar shaft

Mechanism of injury
Direct force to the forearm from a fall or blow.

Clinical presentation
Deformity, pain.

Diagnostics
Physical examination: Swelling, deformity, axial pressure pain, abnormal pronation, and supination.
X-ray examination: X-rays in two planes of the whole of the forearm, so including the elbow and wrist (Fig 6-49).

Classification
None.

Treatment
Conservative treatment: The characteristic of this fracture is that it is incomplete; the periosteum and the cortex are still intact on one side. Bone contact usually remains. On reduction, the radius and the ulna are bent back in the opposite direction to the fractured side. Use the intact periosteum as a hinge. The axis is usually checked with an image intensifier (Fig 6-50). The treatment also consists of a split long-arm cast with the elbow flexed to 90° with three-point pressure for 3–6 weeks.
Surgical treatment: None.

Duration
Fracture takes 4–6 weeks to heal.

Prognosis
Prognosis is good.

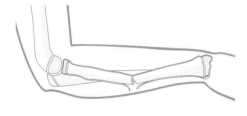

Fig 6-49   Greenstick fracture of the radial shaft in a child.

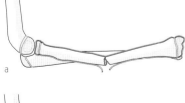

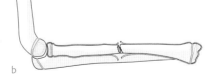

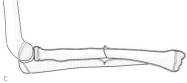

Fig 6-50a–c   Reduction of a greenstick fracture of the radial shaft in a child.

6.20 Distal radial and/or ulnar fractures in children

Mechanism of injury
Direct force to the forearm from a fall or blow, and indirect force by a fall on an outstretched arm.

Clinical presentation
Pain and deformity.

Diagnostics
Physical examination: Loss of function, swelling, pain on palpation, deformity.
X-ray examination: X-rays of the forearm in two planes. Sometimes the fracture is not visible in one view.

Classification
- Torus fracture: slight folding of the bone; the cortex is compressed on one side causing a "fold", the periosteum is intact (Fig 6-51)
- Greenstick fracture (Fig 6-52)
- Complete fracture (Fig 6-53)

Treatment
Conservative treatment: In torus fractures use functional treatment or a dorsal plaster splint for 2 weeks; x-ray check is not necessary. In a greenstick fracture: closed reduction; dorsal forearm splint for 3 weeks.

- With a greenstick fracture there is a risk of redisplacement.

With a complete fracture: closed reduction with the patient under general anesthesia when the aim is to obtain a good radial and ulnar axis. Restoration of full bone contact is not necessary.

- The degree of spontaneous positional correction depends on age, distance of the fracture from the epiphysis, degree of displacement, and direction of the angulation. From age 10 years upward, little spontaneous correction occurs.

Surgical treatment: Only when closed reduction fails or in open fractures use osteosynthesis with plate and screws or intramedullary pins.

Follow-up treatment: Immobilization in a long-arm cast with the elbow flexed to 90° for 6 weeks.

Duration

A torus fracture takes 2–3 weeks to heal; a greenstick fracture, 3–6 weeks; and a complete fracture, 6–8 weeks.

■ Falls are common in children, as are re-fractures, so the immobilization period should not be too short.

Prognosis

Prognosis of a torus fracture and a greenstick fracture is good. After a good reduction, the prognosis of a complex fracture is also good.

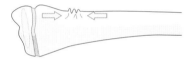

Fig 6-51   Torus fracture of the distal radius in a child.

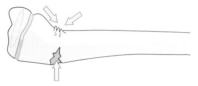

Fig 6-52   Greenstick fracture of the distal radius in a child.

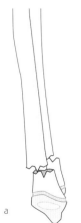

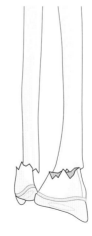

a   b

Fig 6-53a–b   Complete fracture of the distal radius and ulna in a child.

7 Wrist and hand injuries

7.1 Distal radius fractures with displacement/angulation in a dorsal direction

Mechanism of injury
Indirect force caused by a fall on an outstretched hand.

Clinical presentation
Swelling and reduced movement of the wrist. Characteristic clinical deformity often described as "a dinner fork." Deviation of the hand in a radial direction with widening of the wrist contour.

Diagnostics
Physical examination: Pain on palpation, loss of function, and sometimes obvious displacement.
X-ray examination: X-rays of the wrist in two planes. The distal fragment is displaced and angulated dorsally. A fracture of the ulnar styloid process is often present.

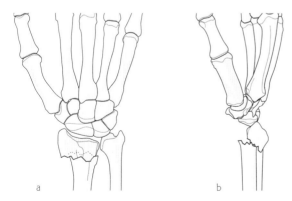

Fig 7-1a–b   Fracture of the distal radius with dorsal displacement: a common fracture pattern.
a AP; b lateral.

Classification

Various classifications exist; the Müller AO Classification is frequently used. Of prognostic importance is:

- Whether the fracture is intraarticular or extraarticular
- Degree of shortening of the radius in relation to the ulna
- Abnormal positioning of carpal bones

Müller AO Classification: 23-A(2–3) (extraarticular) and 23-C(1–3) (intraarticular).

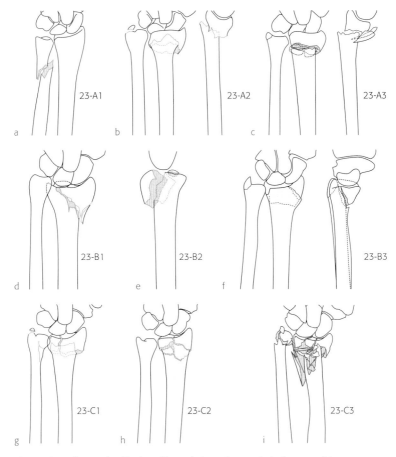

Fig 7-2a–i Müller AO Classification of intraarticular and extraarticular fractures of the distal radius/ulna.

Treatment

Conservative treatment: For marginally displaced fractures or after successful stable reduction use short-arm cast for 4–6 weeks. After reduction, x-ray after 1 week to check position.

Surgical treatment: For severe displacement or if the position obtained after reduction cannot be retained (unstable) use fixation with K-wires (Fig 7-3), osteosynthesis with plate and screws (Fig 7-4), or external fixation.

Duration

Fracture takes 6–9 weeks to heal.
Duration of disability is 3 months.

Prognosis

Prognosis depends on functional demand, restoration of normal anatomy, and identification and treatment of accompanying injury to the ligaments, in particular in relation to the distal radioulnar joint.

- Posttraumatic dystrophy can occur.

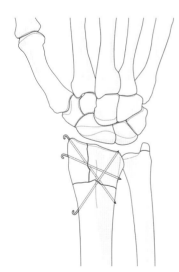

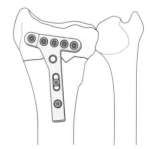

Fig 7-3 Fracture of the distal radius treated with percutaneously inserted K-wires.

Fig 7-4 Fracture of the distal radius treated with plate and screws.

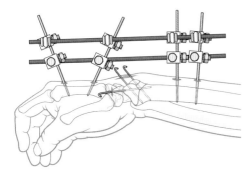

Fig 7-5   Fracture of the distal radius treated with external fixation and percutaneously inserted K-wires.

7.2   Distal radius fractures with displacement/angulation in a palmar direction

Mechanism of injury
A fall on the wrist in palmar flexion or on a supinated forearm whereby an attempt is made to pronate the arm with the hand fixed in dorsiflexion.

Clinical presentation
Pain, swelling of the wrist, reduced movements, and often obvious displacement.

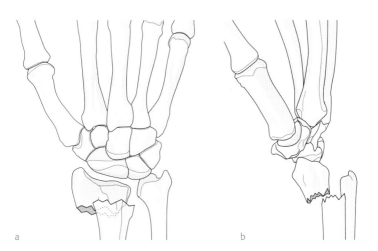

a   b

Fig 7-6a–b   Fracture of the distal radius with palmar displacement. a AP; b lateral.

Diagnostics

Physical examination: "Full" palmar aspect of the wrist, radial deviation of the hand, pain on palpation, and loss of function.

X-ray examination: X-rays of the wrist in two planes—palmar displacement of the distal fracture fragment. The fracture line runs obliquely.

Classification

There are numerous classifications; the Müller AO Classification is most frequently used.

Of importance for the prognosis:

- Is the fracture intraarticular or extraarticular
- Degree of shortening of the radius in relation to the ulna
- Abnormal positioning of carpal bones

Müller AO Classification: 23-A(2–3) (extraarticular) and 23-C(1–3) (intra-articular) (Fig 7-2a–c, g–i).

Treatment

Conservative treatment: In minimally displaced fractures or after successful stable reduction, immobilization in a long-arm cast with the wrist in slight dorsiflexion, the elbow flexed to 90°, and the forearm in supination for 6 weeks.

> ▪ Check for thenar muscle weakness, or impaired sensation, or tingling in the median nerve distribution caused by direct nerve injury by the fracture fragment, or increased pressure in the carpal tunnel.

Surgical treatment: Treatment of choice because these are unstable fractures that redisplace easily; osteosynthesis with plate and screws which are inserted palmarly (Figs 7-3, 7-4).

Duration

Fracture takes 6 weeks to heal.
Duration of disability is on average 3 months.

Prognosis

Prognosis is good if an anatomical reduction is achieved and there is no secondary fracture displacement during healing.

7.3 Partial articular fractures of the distal radius with dorsal fragment

Mechanism of injury

Indirect force caused by a fall on an outstretched arm with an extended wrist.

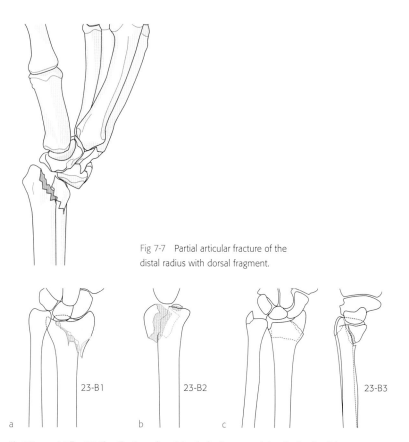

Fig 7-7 Partial articular fracture of the distal radius with dorsal fragment.

23-B1

23-B2

23-B3

a   b   c

Fig 7-8a–c   Müller AO Classification of partial articular fractures of the distal radius/ulna.
a 23-B1: sagittal fragment; b 23-B2: coronal, dorsal rim fragment; c 23-B3: coronal, palmar rim fragment.

Clinical presentation
Pain, swelling, sometimes with obvious deformity of the wrist. The fracture includes the dorsal part of the joint surface.

Diagnostics
Physical examination: Loss of function, pain on palpation.
X-ray examination: X-rays of the wrist in two planes.

Classification
Müller AO Classification: 23-B2.

Treatment
Conservative treatment: Recommended in minimally displaced fractures, with short-arm cast for 4 weeks.

- Beware—this is an unstable fracture with a tendency for secondary displacement.

Surgical treatment: In displaced fractures with dorsal (sub)luxation of the carpus use plate osteosynthesis through a dorsal approach.
Follow-up treatment: Functional.

Duration
Fracture takes 6 weeks to heal.
Duration of disability is usually around 12 weeks.

Prognosis
After anatomical reduction and fixation, the prognosis is good and poor with unreduced incongruity.

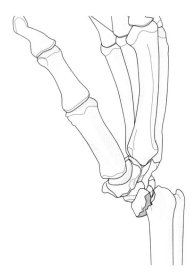

Fig 7-9 Partial articular fracture of the distal radius with palmar fragment.

7.4 Partial articular fractures of the distal radius with palmar fragment

Mechanism of injury
Indirect force caused by a fall on an outstretched arm with an overextended wrist.

Clinical presentation
Pain, swelling, sometimes obvious deformity of the wrist. The fracture includes the palmar aspect of the joint surface.

Diagnostics
Physical examination: Loss of function, pain on palpation.
X-ray examination: X-rays of the wrist in two planes.

Classification
Müller AO Classification: 23-B3.

Treatment
Conservative treatment: Recommended in minimally displaced fractures, use long-arm cast with the forearm in supination for 4 weeks.

■ Beware—this is an unstable fracture with a tendency for secondary displacement.

Surgical treatment: In displaced fractures with palmar (sub)luxation of the carpus use plate osteosynthesis through a palmar approach.
Follow-up treatment: Functional.

Duration
Fracture takes 6 weeks to heal.
Duration of disability is usually about 12 weeks.

Prognosis
After anatomical reduction and fixation the prognosis is good and poor with unreduced incongruity.

7.5   Partial articular fractures of the radius with distal radial styloid fragment

Mechanism of injury
Indirect force caused by forced radial deviation of the wrist, or violent twisting into supination.

Clinical presentation
Pain, swelling. The fracture involves more of the distal radius than the styloid process.

Diagnostics
Physical examination: Loss of function, pain on palpation.
X-ray examination: X-rays of the wrist in two planes.

Classification
Müller AO Classification: 23-B1.

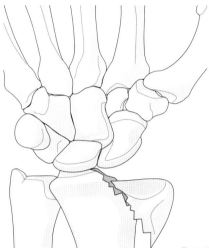

Fig 7-10   Partial articular fracture of the distal radius.

Treatment
Conservative treatment: Use in minimally displaced fractures. Short-arm cast for 4 weeks.

■ This is a potentially unstable fracture due to the accompanying injury to the ligaments.

Surgical treatment: In displaced (intraarticular) fractures, lag screw fixation (often percutaneously) gives more stability than fixation with K-wires.
Follow-up treatment: Short-arm cast if there is any doubt about the stability of the fixation.

Duration
Fracture takes 6 weeks to heal.
Duration of disability is approximately 12 weeks.

Prognosis
After anatomical reduction and fixation the prognosis is good and poor with persistent incongruity.

7.6   Epiphyseal injuries of the distal radius

Mechanism of injury
Indirect trauma caused by a fall on the hand.

Clinical presentation
Pain in the wrist, deformity. This is a frequent injury in children aged between 6 and 10 years.

Diagnostics
Physical examination: Pain on palpation, loss of function, obvious deformity.
X-ray examination: X-rays of the wrist in two planes. There is nearly always dorsal displacement of the epiphysis. Injury to the distal ulna will often accompany injury to the radius. This is sometimes difficult to see on x-ray.

Classification
Epiphysiolysis alone (Salter-Harris type I)—very rare.
Epiphysiolysis with metaphyseal fracture (Salter-Harris type II)—the most common type.
Other types of injuries of the epiphysis are rare.

Treatment
Conservative treatment: Without reduction for minimally displaced fractures; otherwise reduction under local or general anesthesia. Short-arm cast for 3 weeks.
Surgical treatment: Rarely required—only in the irreducible or unstable injury.

Duration
The fracture takes 3–6 weeks to heal depending on the child's age.

Prognosis
Prognosis is good.

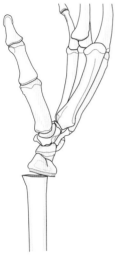

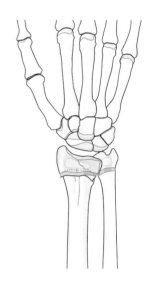

Fig 7-11   Epiphysiolysis of the distal radius, Salter-Harris type I (rare).

Fig 7-12   Epiphysiolysis of the distal radius, Salter-Harris type II.

7.7   Scaphoid fractures

Mechanism of injury
Indirect trauma caused by a fall on the hand with the wrist in hyperextension.

Clinical presentation
Pain, slight swelling. Clinical signs are often minimal, or even absent.

Diagnostics
Physical examination: Pain on movement, swelling, pain on palpation at the level of the anatomical snuffbox, and pain on axial compression of the thumb.
X-ray examination: X-rays in four planes: AP view, 3/4 view with slight dorsiflexion of the wrist, pronated oblique, and lateral view.

■ A scaphoid fracture can be present even though no abnormalities are seen on x-rays. It is therefore recommended that the wrist is immobilized if a scaphoid fracture is strongly suspected, with repeated clinical examination after 10 days and repeated x-rays if necessary. If in doubt, scintigraphy or MRI of the wrist skeleton can be helpful, as the cast does not need to be removed for these investigations.

Classification
According to fracture site (Fig 7-13):
■ Proximal pole
■ Scaphoid waist
■ Tubercle of the scaphoid/distal pole

Treatment
Conservative treatment: Use in fractures with no or minimal displacement. Short-arm cast for 6–12 weeks. It is not necessary to immobilize the whole thumb but in some cases may be more comfortable.

Open surgical treatment: For displaced fractures use reduction and screw fixation.

Percutaneous surgical treatment: Recommended for patients who want to avoid casting.

Duration
The duration of fracture healing depends on the site. The more proximal the location the worse the prognosis and the longer the fracture takes to heal.
■ Fracture of the tubercle: 6 weeks
■ Waist fracture: 6 weeks to 3 months
■ Fracture of the proximal pole: 6 weeks to 3 months with a strong tendency for development of nonunion

The duration of disability varies between 6 weeks and several months, depending on treatment and presence/absence of healing.

Prognosis
After healing, the prognosis is good. Delayed treatment and a proximal fracture are risk factors for poor outcome.

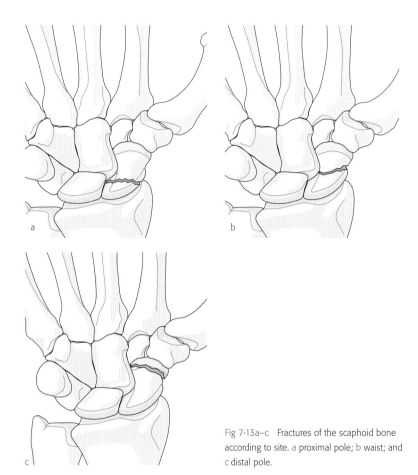

Fig 7-13a–c   Fractures of the scaphoid bone according to site. a proximal pole; b waist; and c distal pole.

7.8   Lunate luxations and perilunate dislocations

Mechanism of injury
Direct high-energy force caused by, for example, a fall from a height on the hand with the wrist in dorsiflexion.

Clinical presentation
Pain, swelling, loss of movement. Many patients complain of altered sensation in the median nerve territory.

Diagnostics
Physical examination: Deformity of the wrist which can easily be missed, as well as restricted range of motion. Altered sensation in the median nerve territory.

X-ray examination: AP view and true lateral view of the wrist. This injury is often missed (up to 20% of cases) because x-ray examination normally focuses on signs of fracture and not on the relationship of the radius to the carpus or the relative arrangement of the carpal bones. Possible helpful additional examinations: MRI and/or CT scans.

■ This injury is common in polytrauma patients, and can be overlooked even in a secondary survey.

■ With lunate luxation the relationship between the radius and the other carpal bones remains intact, while the lunate bone itself is displaced. In a perilunate dislocation the relationship between the radius and the lunate bone remains intact but the other carpal bones are displaced.

Classification
- Isolated damage to ligaments around the lunate bone
- Combined with scaphoid fracture, radial styloid fracture, or capitate fracture
- Palmar displacement
- Axial displacement
- Radiocarpal displacement = perilunate dislocation

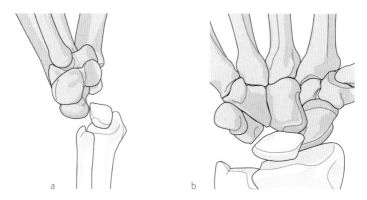

Fig 7-14a–b   Dorsal, perilunate dislocation, the relationship between the lunate and radius is normal; other carpal bones are displaced around the lunate.

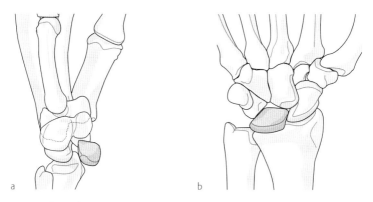

Fig 7-15a–b   Dislocation of the lunate bone. a AP; b lateral.

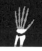

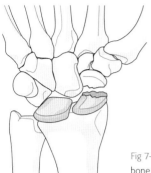

Fig 7-16   Perilunate dislocation with fracture of the scaphoid bone (this is called a "transscaphoid perilunate dislocation").

Treatment

Conservative treatment: Rarely recommended and is reserved for isolated perilunate dislocation. Closed reduction and short-arm cast for 4–6 weeks, with regular x-ray review and conversion to K-wire fixation if displacement occurs.

Surgical treatment: As above, after closed reduction, percutaneous fixation with K-wires. If closed reduction is not possible open reduction and fixation with K-wires is recommended, sometimes with direct ligament repair. When associated with a scaphoid fracture, reduction with operative fixation of the scaphoid fracture.

■ Be alert for injuries to the median nerve.

Follow-up treatment: Short-arm cast for 6–12 weeks.

Duration

Injury takes 6 weeks to heal.
Duration of disability is 6–12 weeks, although permanent stiffness is not unusual.

Prognosis

Prognosis is good.

7.9 Dislocations of the carpometacarpal (CMC) joint of the thumb

Mechanism of injury
Probably longitudinal force with a slight flexion of the MCP joint. With this type of impact, a Bennett fracture is more likely.

Clinical presentation
Pain, swelling, and loss of movement. This injury is rare.

Diagnostics
Physical examination: Swelling of the radial aspect of the hand at the level of the CMC joint. There is some shortening of the thumb, with loss of function and pain on palpation.

X-ray examination: X-rays in two planes. The congruity of the MCP joint is disturbed, proximal displacement of the thumb metacarpal.

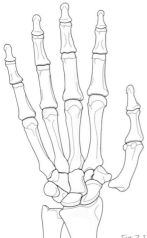

Fig 7-17   Dislocation of the CMC joint of the thumb.

Classification
None.

Treatment
Conservative treatment: Consists of traction and abduction of the thumb with pressure on the base of the thumb metacarpal, then tests the stability after closed reduction. Short-arm cast, including thumb, for 3 weeks.
Surgical treatment: In unstable but congruent joints use temporary transarticular fixation with K-wires after reduction. If unstable and with joint incongruity, exploration to remove any tissue interposition followed by transarticular fixation with K-wires.

Follow-up treatment: Check for redisplacement, short-arm cast, including thumb, for 3 weeks. Remove K-wires after 3 weeks.

Duration
Injury takes 6 weeks to heal.
Duration of disability is 6–8 weeks.

Prognosis
If the joint is congruent, the prognosis is good.

7.10 Basal metacarpal fractures of the thumb

Mechanism of injury
Longitudinal axial force to the thumb.

Clinical presentation
Pain and swelling.

Diagnostics
Physical examination: Loss of function, pain on palpation, and axial pressure.
X-ray examination: X-rays in two planes.
Classification
■ Bennett fracture
■ Rolando fracture (articular T- or Y-shaped fracture)
■ Extraarticular fracture (transverse, oblique, or comminuted epibasal fracture)
■ Injury of the epiphysis, usually Salter-Harris type II

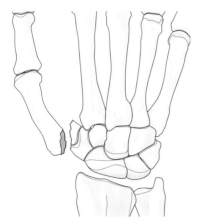

Fig 7-18 Bennett fracture of the base of thumb MC.

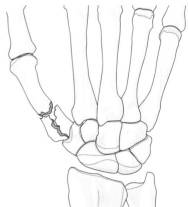

Fig 7-19 Rolando fracture of the base of thumb MC.

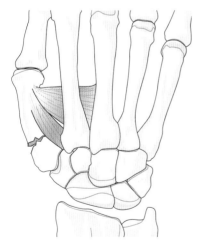

Fig 7-20 Extraarticular fracture of the base of thumb MC with typical ulnar displacement caused by muscle traction.

Treatment

Conservative treatment: For a Rolando fracture with no displacement consists of plaster cast immobilization of the thumb for 4 weeks; for an extraarticular fracture and for injury to the epiphysis, reduction and immobilization in a cast for 3 weeks.

■ Make sure that the MCP joint of the thumb is not overextended in the cast.

Surgical treatment: For a displaced Rolando fracture open reduction and fixation is strongly indicated to restore and maintain articular congruity. As an alternative use ligamentotaxis with external fixation. For injuries to the epiphysis, surgery is indicated in case of inadequate reduction or instability.

Follow-up treatment: For a Rolando fracture early exercises after internal fixation.

Duration

Fracture takes 4–6 weeks to heal.
Duration of disability is 6–8 weeks.

Prognosis

Prognosis is good. For Rolando fractures prognosis depends on the severity of the damage and the accuracy of reduction.

7.11 Fracture subluxations of the carpometacarpal joint of the thumb

Mechanism of injury

Longitudinal axial force to the adducted thumb.

Clinical presentation

Swelling and pain on moving the thumb.

Diagnostics

Physical examination: Loss of function, pain on axial pressure.

X-ray examination: X-rays in two planes. The thumb metacarpal is displaced proximally; part of the epiphysis of the thumb metacarpal with a segment of the articular surface retains a normal relationship with the trapezium bone/ multiangular bone.

Classification
None.

Treatment
Conservative treatment: There is no consensus on how to treat this injury. Supporters of a conservative approach note that patients have few symptoms from a fracture that has healed with a degree of displacement. Treatment consists of closed reduction and plaster cast, including the thumb.

■ Make sure that the MCP joint of the thumb is not overextended in the cast.

Others prefer reduction and fixation to correct incongruity of the joint, highlighting the increased incidence of x-ray changes of arthrosis in persistent incongruity.

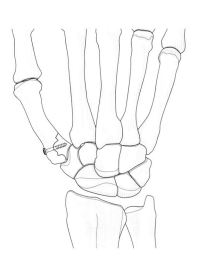

Fig 7-21   Bennett fracture treated with lag screw.

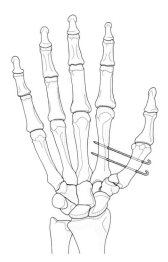

Fig 7-22   Bennett fracture treated with K-wires between thumb and index MCs.

Surgical treatment: In a new injury closed reduction can be performed, aided by an image intensifier. Percutaneous fixation with K-wires either between the thumb and index metacarpals or transarticularly (CMC). If reduction is inadequate, open reduction and fixation, eg, with a screw or K-wire that holds the thumb and index metacarpals together.

Follow-up treatment: After surgical treatment with screw fixation, exercises can be started early. After percutaneous K-wire fixation, remove wires at 4–6 weeks and mobilize. With conservative treatment, short-arm cast, including thumb, for 4 weeks.

Duration
Injury takes 6 weeks to heal.
Duration of disability is 6–8 weeks.

Prognosis
Prognosis is good.

7.12   Dislocations of the carpometacarpal joints (CMC) II–V

Mechanism of injury
Direct axial high-energy force to the hand.

Clinical presentation
Pain and swelling. This injury is not common and is mainly seen in polytrauma patients. The carpometacarpal joints II and III are fixed and IV and V have a restricted range of motion. Isolated injury to the carpometacarpal joints IV and V is seen most frequently after a punching injury.

Diagnostics
Physical examination: Diffuse swelling around area of injury, local pain on palpation, and pain on axial pressure.
X-ray examination: X-rays in three planes; AP, true lateral view, and 20° pronated view.

Classification
- According to direction of displacement: dorsal or palmar
- True luxation or fracture luxation

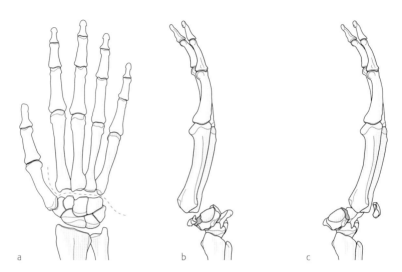

Fig 7-23a–c   Fracture subluxation of carpometacarpal joints II–V. a AP view of plane of dislocation;
b Palmar dislocation of carpometacarpal joints; c Dorsal dislocation of carpometacarpal joints.

Treatment
Conservative treatment: Traction and local pressure to achieve reduction.
Short-arm cast, leaving the MCP joints free, for 3 weeks.
Surgical treatment: For unstable fractures (which is the usual situation) use
closed reduction and percutaneous K-wire fixation. In fractures of the base of
the metacarpals use screw fixation after open reduction if the bone fragments
are of sufficient size. For comminuted fractures of the base use fixation with
plate and screws to bridge the CMC joints.

Duration
Injury takes 4 weeks to heal.
Duration of disability is 6–8 weeks.

Prognosis
If the reduction is adequate, the prognosis is good. Posttraumatic arthrosis
is not uncommon some time after healing of a highly comminuted articular
injury.

7.13 Fracture subluxations of the carpometacarpal (CMC) joint V

Mechanism of injury
Longitudinal force, often caused by catching the little finger in something.

Clinical presentation
Swelling and pain when moving the little finger.

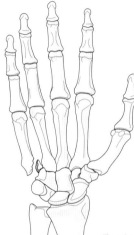

Fig 7-24   Fracture subluxation of CMC joint V.

Diagnostics
Physical examination: Loss of function, local tenderness, and pain on axial pressure.
X-ray examination: X-rays in three planes. Metacarpal V is displaced proximally; part of the joint retains a normal relation with the hamate bone.

Classification
None.

Treatment
Conservative treatment: The fifth CMC joint is the second most mobile after the thumb. Good reduction in longitudinal traction and with local pressure is necessary. Use an image intensifier. Short-arm cast for 3 weeks.

- Risk of redisplacement.

Surgical treatment: If insufficient reduction is achieved or if redisplacement occurs, reduction and percutaneous K-wire fixation is indicated.

Follow-up treatment: Short-arm cast for 3 weeks, then remove K-wires.

Duration
Fracture takes 6 weeks to heal.
Duration of disability is 6–8 weeks.

Prognosis
Prognosis is good.

7.14   Fractures of the shaft of metacarpals II–V

Mechanism of injury
Direct force from a blow or fall. Forced rotation.

Clinical presentation
Swelling and pain.

Diagnostics
Physical examination: Loss of function of the hand, sometimes rotational abnormalities or shortening of the finger, local tenderness, and pain on axial pressure.

X-ray examination: X-rays of the hand in two planes.

Classification
- **Transverse fracture:** result of direct force
- **Oblique fracture:** rotational injury of the finger
- **Spiral fracture:** rotational injury of the finger
- **Comminuted fracture:** result of considerable force

  - Transverse and especially comminuted fractures can be the result of considerable axial force that also leads to severe soft-tissue injuries and sometimes an open fracture. These injuries are often associated with other skeletal trauma.

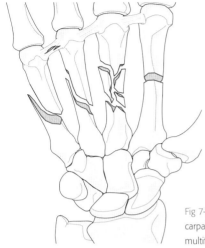

Fig 7-25 Different types of fracture of the meta-carpal shaft: fifth, spiral; fourth, long oblique; third, multifragmentary; and second, transverse.

Treatment

Conservative treatment: Only used in transverse fractures if there is minimal displacement and if the condition of the soft tissues permits. Transverse fractures tend toward dorsal angulation; the more proximal the fracture, the more obvious the angulation. After conservative treatment displacement often remains causing a noticeable lump to develop. With an oblique or spiral fracture, shortening is less of a problem unless the fracture occurs in a border metacarpal (II or V), but a rotational abnormality can occur. Check position of nails. Short-arm cast with the hand in a functional position for 3 weeks.

Surgical treatment: Often indicated for multiple fractures. Osteosynthesis of one or more metacarpals. Surgery is also indicated for spiral fractures with rotation and in comminuted fractures because of damage to soft tissues. The treatment is carried out using K-wires, or a plate and screws.

- Fractures of metacarpals II and V tend to be associated with shortening and rotation.

Follow-up treatment: Depending on the stability achieved, use short-arm cast with the hand in a functional position for 3 weeks, then start exercises as soon as possible.

Duration
Fracture takes 6–8 weeks to heal.
Duration of disability largely depends on damage to soft tissues.

Prognosis
Prognosis is good.

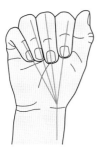

Fig 7-26   Assessment of rotation at the level of metacarpal fractures. Check position of nails, fingers point to one point over the scaphoid tubercle.

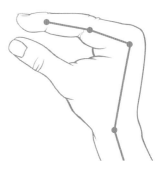

Fig 7-27   Functional position of the hand to minimize stiffness during immobilization.

7.15   Subcapital (neck) fractures of metacarpals II–V

Mechanism of injury
Direct axial force from a blow with the fist or other impact.

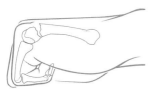

Fig 7-28   Subcapital fracture of a metacarpal bone with typical displacement.

Clinical presentation
Swelling, pain, obvious deformity.

Diagnostics
Physical examination: Loss of function, pain on axial pressure, the knuckle of the broken metacarpal is displaced and is noted to have "dropped" on making a fist. The head may be palpable in the palm. This injury usually occurs with the metacarpal V.

X-ray examination: X-rays of the hand in two planes.

Classification
None.

Treatment
Conservative treatment: The following angulation can be accepted as a guide, although individual decisions will be made in each case:

- Metacarpal II–III: 15°
- Metacarpal IV: 20°
- Metacarpal V: 30°

If the angulation is too great and the head is displaced, this can cause pain in the palm of the hand on forceful gripping and reduced pinch strength.

A nondisplaced fracture with acceptable angulation is treated functionally. Other fractures are reduced and immobilized in a palmar plaster splint in a 90°/0°/0° position, and strapped to the adjacent finger for 3 weeks.

Surgical treatment: Only used with severe displacement or instability, with percutaneous or intramedullary K-wire fixation in combination with a plaster splint for 3 weeks.

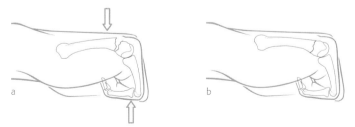

Fig 7-29a–b   Reduction of a subcapital fracture of metacarpal V. a Reduction technique.
b Reduced fracture.

Duration
Fracture takes 3–6 weeks to heal.
Duration of disability is also 3–6 weeks.

Prognosis
Prognosis is good.

7.16 Dislocations of the metacarpophalangeal (MCP) joint of the thumb

Mechanism of injury
Generally caused by overextension of the MCP joint; eg, a fall on the hand.

Clinical presentation
Pain, deformity of the thumb.

Diagnostics
Physical examination: The thumb is shortened in hyperextension, swelling of the thenar muscles.
X-ray examination: X-rays in two planes (Fig 7-30); sometimes a sesamoid bone is visible in the joint gap indicating displacement of the flexor tendon.

Treatment
Conservative treatment: Reduction is more often successful when the flexor tendon is not displaced. After reduction, the stability should be tested as well as the range of passive movements of the joint. Short-arm splint, including thumb, for 3 weeks.
Surgical treatment: In cases of instability or if reduction is not achieved, remove any tissue interposition (palmar plate, tendon of the flexor pollicis longus muscle).
Follow-up treatment: Splinting for 3 weeks.

Duration
Injury takes 6–8 weeks to heal.
Duration of disability is 8–10 weeks.

Prognosis
Prognosis is good.

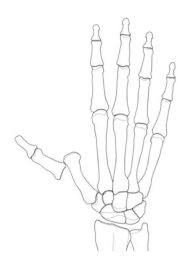

Fig 7-30   Dislocation of the MCP joint of the thumb.

7.17   Ulnar collateral ligament injuries of the metacarpophalangeal (MCP) joint of the thumb

Mechanism of injury
Forced abduction of an extended thumb, classically when skiing.

Clinical presentation
Pain, local swelling; the joint is painful when pinching or grasping and the thumb is generally weak.

Diagnostics
Physical examination: Pain on palpation at the ulnar aspect of the MCP joint. Abnormal abduction of the thumb when the joint is in slight flexion. Instability in extension is a sign that the palmar plate is also torn.
X-ray examination: X-rays in two planes (Fig 7-32). Bone avulsion can be present at the base of the proximal phalanx.

- Stress x-rays are rarely indicated.

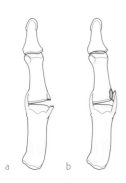

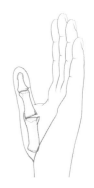

Fig 7-31a–b Ulnar ligament injuries of the MCP joint of the thumb.
a Ligament injury only; b avulsion fracture.

Fig 7-32 Position of the hand for taking a good AP view of the MCP joint of the thumb.

Classification
With or without bony avulsion of the proximal phalanx.

Treatment
Conservative treatment: For bone avulsion with a small, minimally displaced fragment; immobilization of the MCP joint in flexion in a cast for 3 weeks.
Surgical treatment: For displaced avulsion fragments or isolated ligamentous injury.
Follow-up treatment: Plaster cast with the joint in flexion for 3 weeks after bony injury; 6 weeks after soft-tissue repair.

Duration
Injury takes 3–6 weeks to heal.
Duration of disability is also 3–6 weeks.

Prognosis
Prognosis is good with regard to stability and pain. Generally, there is some loss of flexion but this does not produce any functional restrictions.

7.18 Subluxations/dislocations of the metacarpophalangeal (MCP) joints of digits II–V

Mechanism of injury
Catching the finger in something, or overextension.

Clinical presentation
Subluxation or dislocation of the little finger is most common; deformity, pain. This injury is often associated with open wounds.

Diagnostics
Physical examination: Inability to move MCP joint, deformity.

■ A wound on the flexor surface of the finger or between the fourth and fifth metacarpal shafts may indicate joint disruption.

X-ray examination: X-rays in two planes; incongruity of the affected joint.

■ If in doubt about the congruity of a joint, compare it with other MCP joints.

Classification
Simple: There is no soft-tissue interposition.
Complex: The metacarpal head tears the palmar plate longitudinally and passes through the tear. Attempts at closed reduction by traction are often fruitless as the tear tightens with ligamentotaxis.

Treatment
Conservative treatment: After closed reduction, ensure that MCP joint can move freely (passively); also perform an x-ray check.
Surgical treatment: Required if closed reduction is unsuccessful. Exploration from the palmar surface is necessary to remedy the soft-tissue interposition. Great care must be taken to avoid digital nerves which will lie displaced just under the skin surface and are vulnerable to injury. Use of a tourniquet is essential.
Follow-up treatment: Palmar splint for 3 weeks.

Duration
Injury takes 6 weeks to heal.
Duration of disability is 6–8 weeks, depending on the patient's occupation.

Prognosis
Prognosis is good.

7.19   Fractures of the base of the proximal phalanx of the finger

Mechanism of injury
Direct force caused by a fall, a heavy object, or twisting force.

Clinical presentation
Pain, swelling, deformity. This injury is more common than a fracture of the middle phalanx and less common than a fracture of the distal phalanx.

Diagnostics
Physical examination: Pain on palpation, loss of function. On flexion of MCP joints and flexion of proximal interphalangeal (PIP) joints, rotational abnormalities become visible.
X-ray examination: X-rays in two planes, centered on the injured digit.

- Usually an x-ray is taken of the hand without a true lateral view. This means the degree of angulation is difficult to assess.

- On evaluating the AP view of one finger, it is difficult to establish abnormalities of the longitudinal axis. This abnormality is more obvious on physical examination.

Classification
- **Transverse fracture:** nearly always the result of a direct force; an unstable fracture
- **Oblique fracture:** with a tendency for rotation
- **Comminuted fracture:** as a result of considerable direct force

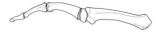

Fig 7-33   Transverse fracture of the base of the proximal phalanx of the finger.

Treatment

Conservative treatment: Depends on the displacement and stability, and is used in fractures with no or minimal displacement, eg, by fixation to the adjacent finger with strapping. This maintains the anatomical position; exercises can then be started. Treatment with a plaster cast is also possible. Displaced fractures are reduced, after which the stability is tested. Immobilization in a cast is only indicated for a stable reduction with MCP joints flexed to at least 70° and PIP joints not flexed more than 15–20°. Oblique fractures are hardly ever stable after closed reduction and tend to displace.

Surgical treatment: Used for unstable fractures, especially if a rotational displacement is anticipated for open fractures and for fractures with accompanying injuries to tendon and neurological injuries.

Follow-up treatment: Physical examination and an x-ray check are certainly necessary if there is any doubt about the stability after reduction. An advantage of surgical treatment is that exercises can be started soon after stable fixation.

■ Contractures tend to occur in PIP joints if they are immobilized in flexion.

Duration
Fracture takes 4–6 weeks to heal.
Duration of disability depends highly on the patient's occupation.

Prognosis
The prognosis is mainly determined by the degree of restriction in the range of motion of the PIP joint.

7.20 Intraarticular fractures of the interphalangeal joints (condylar fractures)

Mechanism of injury
Forced ulnar/radial deviation of the finger (catching in something).

Clinical presentation
Pain, swelling around the joint.

Diagnostics
Physical examination: Symptoms can be similar to those of a dislocation.

■ Axial and rotational abnormalities are suggestive of a significant injury.

X-ray examination: X-rays in two planes, centered on the injured finger.

Classification

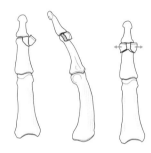

Fig 7-34   Intraarticular fractures of the phalangeal condyles of the finger.

Classification of this injury is dependent on two factors—whether or not the joint is dislocated/subluxed and what the fracture pattern is.
Fracture configuration: Articular fractures can be unicondylar or bicondylar. Bicondylar fractures are either T- or Y-shaped.

Treatment
Conservative treatment: For minimally displaced fractures use immobilization in plaster cast in the functional position. For displacement and instability, circle traction according to Schenk is one reliable method.

■ The treatment is often started late because of delay in presentation or inappropriate assessment.

Surgical treatment: Axial/rotational abnormalities or subluxation lead to serious problems. The treatment consists of open reduction and fixation with a lag screw or K-wires because the fracture is unstable and the articular surface is disrupted.
Follow-up treatment: Depending on the stability achieved use plaster cast for 3 weeks, or early exercises.

Duration
Fracture heals in 3–6 weeks.
Duration of disability can be several months. These injuries often require intensive physical therapy.

Prognosis
Prognosis for significantly displaced or comminuted fractures is poor; restrictions usually remain in the range of motion.

7.21   Fractures of the middle phalanx of the finger

Mechanism of injury
Direct force caused by a fall or blow from a heavy object, or twisting force.

Clinical presentation
Pain, swelling, deformity, soft-tissue injury. Fractures of the proximal and distal phalanx are more common.

Diagnostics
Physical examination: Loss of function, pain on palpation and axial pressure, obvious deformity.
X-ray examination: X-rays in two planes centered on the injured finger.

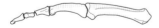

Fig 7-35   Transverse fracture of the middle phalanx of the finger.

Classification
- Transverse fracture
- Oblique fracture (long or short oblique)
- Comminuted fracture

Treatment
Conservative treatment: Depending on the displacement and stability, use reduction and immobilization in a palmar splint with the hand in a 90°/0°/0° position.

■ The middle phalanx is almost completely composed of cortical bone. Reduction should be carried out carefully to spare the periosteum.

Surgical treatment: Often indicated in cases of inadequate reduction or with instability. Use fixation with K-wires, lag screws, mini plates, or external fixation.

Duration
Fracture takes 3–6 weeks to heal.
Duration of disability is 6 weeks to several months.

Prognosis
If reduction is inadequate, the prognosis is poor. When displacement remains, there is a tendency for adhesions or tenosynovitis of the flexor tendon sheath.

7.22   Fractures of the distal phalanx of the finger

Mechanism of injury
Direct force caused by, eg, a heavy object or a jamming injury. Often associated with partial amputation.

Clinical presentation
Fractures of the distal phalanx are often associated with wounds (open fractures), damage to the nail bed, displacement of the nail plate, or a subungual hematoma.

Diagnostics
Physical examination: Pain, swelling, local tenderness, subungual hematoma nail deformities.
X-ray examination: X-rays in two planes centered on the injured finger.

Classification
- Longitudinal fracture (wedge fracture)
- Fracture at the level of the (old) epiphysis: this injury often occurs in children
- Comminuted fracture (often called a "tuft" fracture)

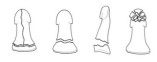

Fig 7-36   Fractures of the distal phalanx of the finger.

Treatment

Conservative treatment: Especially directed to injuries of soft tissues; eg, with decompression of the painful subungual hematoma with a red-hot paperclip or sterile hypodermic needle.

Surgical treatment: Usually for cleaning the soft-tissue injury or for significant fracture displacement by reduction and fixation with K-wires.

■ Interposition of the nail bed results in a poorly healing wound, osteitis of the distal phalanx, and malformation of the nail. When this occurs at the physis, it is called a "Seymour fracture." The interposition needs to be remedied, after which the fracture can be reduced and fixed with K-wires. If the nail has displaced from under the nail fold, it must be replaced and usually secured.

Duration

Fracture takes 3–6 weeks to heal.
Duration of disability is also 3–6 weeks.

Prognosis

Prognosis is mainly determined by soft-tissue injuries.

7.23   Subluxations and dislocations of the interphalangeal joints of the finger

Mechanism of injury

Direct axial or angulatory force rotation.

Clinical presentation

Pain, deformity.

Fig 7-37   Dislocation of the distal interphalangeal joint in the finger.

Diagnostics
Physical examination: Swelling, the interphalangeal joint is flexed, movement is painful. There is sometimes a wound.

■ Diagnosis is often missed.

X-ray examination: X-rays in two planes. The lateral view usually shows dorsal displacement of the distal phalanx. Bone avulsion can occur on the dorsal or palmar surface. A dorsal avulsion represents an extensor tendon injury and joint subluxation is often screen. A palmar avulsion represents a palmar plate injury.

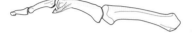

Fig 7-38 Injury of the palmar plate with bone avulsion of the interphalangeal joint of the finger.

Classification
None.

Treatment
Conservative treatment: Closed reduction, splint for 3 weeks (or 6 weeks if associated with a mallet finger).

■ An x-ray check of the position of the joint after reduction is necessary because reduction is sometimes incomplete due to interposition of the palmar plate, the long flexor tendon, or a bone fragment.

Surgical treatment: Transarticular fixation with a K-wire is required in unstable or delayed cases.

Duration
Fracture takes 2–4 weeks to heal.
Duration of disability is also 4–6 weeks.

Prognosis
Prognosis is good.

7.24 Mallet finger

Mechanism of injury
Sudden abrupt flexion of the extended distal interphalangeal (DIP) joint.

Clinical presentation
The fingertip is flexed and cannot be actively straightened out. This injury is common in ball sports; it is also known as the bed-making finger because it frequently occurs in middle-aged and elderly patients as they tuck bed sheets under the mattress.

Diagnostics
Physical examination: Restricted active extension; the finger can be fully extended passively. Minimal swelling, minimal pain.
X-ray examination: X-rays in two planes to show an avulsion fracture of the distal phalanx.

- Beware of subluxation.

Classification
- True tendon rupture, without skeletal trauma
- Tendon rupture with bone avulsion

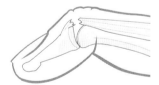
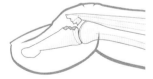

Fig 7-39   Mallet finger with tendon rupture.   Fig 7-40   Mallet finger with bone avulsion.

Treatment
Conservative treatment: A splint using the device described by Stack in hyperextension for 6 weeks (Fig 7-41).
Surgical treatment: Osteosynthesis is only used for a large fracture fragment with subluxation of the DIP joint.

Duration
Injury takes 6 weeks to heal.

Prognosis

Active hyperextension of DIP joint nearly always remains restricted by 20°
or 30°.

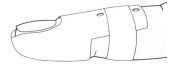

Fig 7-41   Mallet finger treated with a Stack splint.

8   Spine and pelvic injuries

8   Spine and pelvic injuries

8.1   Fracture/dislocation of cervical spine

Mechanism of injury
Diving into shallow water, motor vehicle injury, or hanging.

Clinical presentation
Neck pain and torticollis. Inability to lift the head.

May have neurological deficit of the arms and/or legs. For grading see ASIA (American Spinal Injury Association) scale (Table 8-1).

■ Attention: Regardless of any impression about the severity of cervical trauma or possible comorbidities a predefined diagnostic algorithm must be used for evaluation of the cervical spine in all high-energy trauma patients.

■ Be alert for cervical spine injury in polytrauma, coma, intoxication, or head and facial injuries when physical signs may be overlooked or difficult to obtain.

Diagnostics
X-ray examination: For decision-making use algorithm (Fig 8-1).

Neurological evaluation:
■ **Sensory function:** Examine all dermatomes, starting from cranial to caudal, and both the right and left sides. Mark the borders of sensory function change (Fig 8-2).
■ **Motor function:** Should be examined in the upper and lower extremity, noting the level of motor function change (Table 8-1).

The bulbocavernosus reflex should be tested. A negative sign means the patient is in spinal shock, which is a temporally physiological dysfunction of the spinal cord without any sensory or motor function below the injury. Usually the resolution of the spinal shock occurs between 24 and 48 hours, and can be diagnosed when the bulbocavernosus reflex begins to function again.

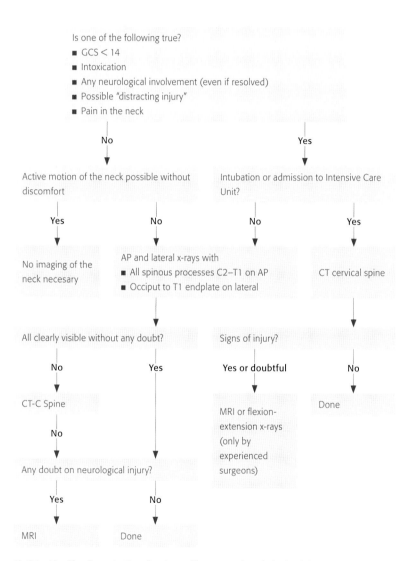

Is one of the following true?
- GCS < 14
- Intoxication
- Any neurological involvement (even if resolved)
- Possible "distracting injury"
- Pain in the neck

No

Yes

Active motion of the neck possible without discomfort

Intubation or admission to Intensive Care Unit?

Yes

No

No

Yes

No imaging of the neck necesary

AP and lateral x-rays with
- All spinous processes C2–T1 on AP
- Occiput to T1 endplate on lateral

CT cervical spine

All clearly visible without any doubt?

Signs of injury?

No

Yes

Yes or doubtful

No

CT-C Spine

MRI or flexion-extension x-rays (only by experienced surgeons)

Done

No

Any doubt on neurological injury?

Yes

No

MRI

Done

Fig 8-1 Algorithm for evaluation of patients with suspected cervical spine injury.

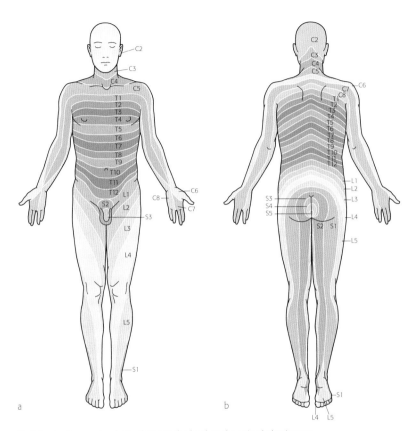

Fig 8-2a–b Sensory levels in relation to the level on the spinothalamic tract.

American Spinal Injury Associaten (ASIA) Score

A	Complete	No motor or sensory function is preserved including the sacral segments S4/5.
B	Incomplete	Sensory but not motor function is preserved below the neurological level and includes the sacral segments S4/5.
C	Incomplete	Motor function is preserved below the neurological level, and more than half of key muscles below the neurological level have a muscle grade less than 3.
D	Incomplete	Motor function is preserved below the neurological level, and at least half of key muscles below the neurological level have a muscle grade of 3 or more.
E	Normal	Motor and sensory functions are normal.

Muscle grading

0	Total paralysis
1	Palpable or visible contraction
2	Active movement, full range of motion, gravity eliminated
3	Active movement, full range of motion, against gravity
4	Active movement, full range of motion, against gravity and provides some resistance
5	Active movement, full range of motion, against gravity and provides normal resistance

Motor function levels (intact)

C5	Elbow flexion
C6	Wrist extension
C7	Elbow extension
C8	Flexion of the third finger
T1	Abduction of the fifth finger
L2	Hip flexion
L3	Knee extension
L4	Dorsiflexion of the foot
L5	Extension of the hallux
S1	Plantar flexion of the foot

Table 8-1 Testing of neurological function.

Treatment
Specific fractures are covered in the respective chapter.

■ For patients with neurological abnormalities attention should be paid to bladder control and prevention of decubitus (pressure sores) from the time of initial injury.

■ The psychological effects of neck injuries with neurological deficit are vast. Patients should be given full and honest information regarding therapeutic possibilities and prognosis.

Duration
Spinal cord shock lasts 24–48 hours.

Prognosis
Prognosis is determined by the degree of neurological involvement.

8.2   Soft-tissue injury to cervical spine

Mechanism of injury
Forced acceleration/deceleration or fall on the head.

Clinical presentation
Neck pain increasing with movement.

Diagnostics
Physical examination: Diffuse pain on palpation with muscle spasms.
X-ray examination: See algorithm on Fig 8-1.

Classification
None.

Treatment
Reassure the patient and administer analgesics, gradually reducing the dose over 2 weeks.

Duration
Injury takes 2–3 weeks to heal.
Duration of disability is also 2–3 weeks.

Prognosis
Prognosis is good; pain starts to subside after a few days.

8.3 Whiplash injury

Mechanism of injury
Head-to-tail collision: probably with more translation than flexion/extension of the neck.

Clinical presentation
There is often a symptom-free interval of a few hours to weeks. Neck pain is reported without any objective evidence of damage to the cervical spine. Neuropsychological symptoms include dizziness, concentration and memory problems, sleep disorder, and/or headache.

Diagnostics
Physical examination: No specific findings.
X-ray examination: Acute examination (see algorithm on Fig 8-1). X-rays including flexion extension to be repeated after 1–3 weeks if necessary. MRI provides no additional information.

Treatment
Conservative treatment: Patient education; if time is taken to explain the injury to the patient and show understanding and empathy, the injury or severity of injury may be prevented or diminished. Treatment can also include an exercise program with slowly increasing activities (graded activity) and/or analgesics that are diminished over time. There is no evidence that a soft collar provides any benefit.

   ■ The chronic manifestation of whiplash can be part of posttraumatic stress syndrome or deconditioning syndrome, with persistent pain and dysfunction.

Surgical treatment: No indications.

Prognosis
Approximately 25% of patients recover within 2 weeks, 50% have persisting mild symptoms, 15% continue to have serious problems but remain functional and at work, and 10% have permanent symptoms with disability.

8.4   Subluxation of facet joints

Mechanism of injury
Forced acceleration/deceleration, eg, from a head-to-tail collision.

Clinical presentation
Neck pain and torticollis. This is a rare injury, usually seen in young patients.

Diagnostics
Physical examination: Pain on palpation and torticollis.
X-ray examination: The lateral view shows an abnormal positioning of the facet joints with respect to each other without a frank dislocation.

Classification
None.

Treatment
Immobilization in a rigid neck collar. As pain subsides, start functional treatment.

Duration
Injury takes 3–6 weeks to heal.
Duration of disability also lasts for 3–6 weeks.

Prognosis
Prognosis is good because there are no injuries to the ligaments.

- Consider possibility of a whiplash injury.

8.5 Dislocation of facet joints

Mechanism of injury
Flexion-distraction injury from forced acceleration/deceleration or fall on the head.

Clinical presentation
Neck pain with marked muscle spasm and possible torticollis.

Diagnostics
Physical examination: Neck pain with hypertonic musculature. Torticollis can occur, sometimes linked to neurological deficit.

- This injury is unstable in flexion.

X-ray examination: See algorithm on Fig 8-1. With unilateral dislocation of facet joints, the superior spinous process points to the involved side on AP view. The lateral x-ray shows ±25% anterior displacement of the vertebral body at the level of the dislocation in relation to the inferior vertebral body. With bilateral dislocation of facet joints, a widening of the interspinal space is seen on AP view. The lateral view shows ±50% anterior displacement of the vertebral body at the level of dislocation in relation to the inferior vertebral body (Fig 8-3).
MRI is indicated to exclude traumatic herniated disc.

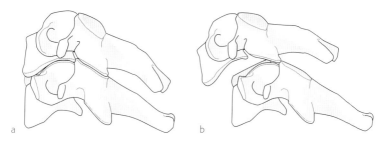

Fig 8-3a–b   a Normal lateral alignment of two adjacent cervical vertebrae. b A lateral view of bilateral dislocation of facet joints of the cervical vertebrae.

Classification

- Unilateral dislocation
- Bilateral dislocation

Treatment

Conservative treatment: Closed reduction by gradually increasing traction. Then immobilization in a rigid neck collar or with halo vest. An associated facet fracture may block reduction by closed techniques. Such fractures may also cause instability following reduction. Surgery is indicated in both cases.

Surgical treatment: Closed/open reduction and spondylodesis (anterior or posterior).

Duration

Injury takes 8–12 weeks to heal.
Duration of disability lasts several months.

Prognosis

Prognosis for this spinal column injury is good; if present, the neurological deficit determines the prognosis.

8.6   C1–C2 dislocation

Mechanism of injury

High-energy trauma, fall from height, or hanging.

Clinical presentation

Varies from neck pain to a dramatic clinical picture with complete paraplegia and respiratory insufficiency resulting in death.

- This is potentially an extremely unstable injury.

Diagnostics

Physical examination: Neck pain, few conspicuous local abnormalities. Signs of any accompanying spinal cord injury will be prominent.

X-ray examination: See algorithm on Fig 8-1.

Classification
- Type A: anterior dislocation with injury of the transverse ligament
- Type B: anterior dislocation with fracture of the odontoid process (dens)
- Type C: dorsal dislocation
- Type D: rotatory dislocation

> ■ In type A, the distance between the posterior aspect of the anterior arch of C1 and the anterior aspect of the odontoid process is increased on the lateral view. This distance is normally ±3 mm in adults and ±5 mm in children.

Treatment
Conservative treatment: Closed reduction with the patient under general anesthesia. Then immobilization in a halo vest.

Surgical treatment: Screw fixation of the odontoid process in type B or spondylodesis C1–C2 may be used.

Duration
Lasting 8–12 weeks.

Prognosis
Prognosis is good if there is no accompanying neurological deficit.

8.7   C1 fracture (Jefferson fracture)

Mechanism of injury
Axial loading force. Diving into shallow water.

Clinical presentation
Pain high in the neck and torticollis. Neurological deficit is rarely present.

Diagnostics
Physical examination: Hypertonic musculature, torticollis. Few specific symptoms.

X-ray examination: X-rays of the cervical spine in two planes, including the odontoid process. On a standard x-ray, the fracture may not be clearly visible. CT scan is therefore indicated.

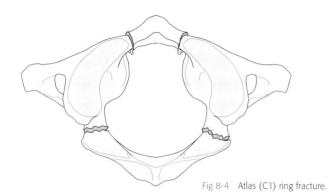

Fig 8-4   Atlas (C1) ring fracture.

Classification
Depending on the integrity of the transverse ligament. If transverse ligament is injured, C1–C2 instability may result.

Treatment
Rigid neck collar or halo vest in case of injury to the transverse ligament.

Duration
Injury takes 8–12 weeks to heal.
Duration of disability is 3–4 months.

Prognosis
Prognosis is good if there is no neurological deficit. In the long term C1–C2 joint arthrosis may follow.

8.8   Arch of C2 fracture (traumatic lysis or "Hangman's" fracture)

Mechanism of injury
Axial loading force, fall on the head, or hanging.

Clinical presentation
Pain high in the neck and torticollis.

Diagnostics
Physical examination: Hypertonic musculature and torticollis. No specific symptoms.
X-ray examination: X-rays of the cervical spine in two planes, including a view of the odontoid process. Fractures of the arch of C2 may not be visible on conventional x-rays. CT scan is thus indicated.

Classification (Levine and Edwards)
Type 1:   nondisplaced, C2–C3 intervertebral disc intact (Fig 8-5a)
Type 1A: involvement of one pars interarticularis, extending anterior into the body of the contralateral side, promoting an oblique displacement
Type 2:   flexion-type injury with C2–C3 displacement, translation >3mm, disruption of C2–C3 disc
Type 2A: flexion-distraction injury with severe C2 angulation over C3, avulsion of entire C2–C3 intervertebral disc, and injury of the posterior longitudinal ligament (Fig 8-5b)
Type 3:   dislocation of C2–C3 joint facets with severe angulation and translation displacement

Treatment
Depends on stability of the injury.
Types 1 and 2 are usually stable and require a rigid collar immobilization for 6 weeks.
Types 2A and 3 injuries are unstable, and should be treated by halo vest or C2–C3 posterior fusion.

Duration
Injury takes 6–8 weeks to heal.
Duration of disability is 3–4 months.

Prognosis
Prognosis is good if there is no neurological deficit.

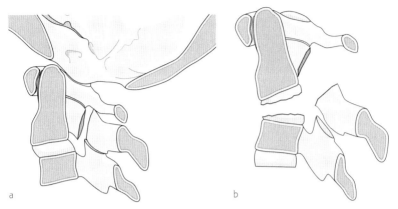

a   b

Fig 8-5a–b   a Type 1 fracture of the arch of C2. b Type 2A flexion distraction injury of C2.

8.9   Odontoid process fracture (dens)

Mechanism of injury
Axial loading force, fall on the front or back of the head.

Clinical presentation
Pain high in the neck and torticollis. There is usually no neurological deficit.

Diagnostics
Physical examination: Hypertonic musculature and torticollis. Few specific symptoms.
X-ray examination: See algorithm on Fig 8-1. Usually visible on x-rays of the cervical spine in two planes, including a view of the odontoid process. For an exact assessment, CT scan is essential.

■ Odontoid fractures are frequently associated with a second injury at the level of the cervicothoracic vertebral junction.

Classification

The Anderson classification distinguishes three types:

Type I: oblique fracture through the apex of the odontoid process. This is an avulsion of the alar ligaments (Fig 8-6a). May be associated with occiputocervical injuries.

Type II: transverse fracture at the level of what was the epiphysis (Fig 8-6b)

Type III: transverse fracture through part of the vertebral body, extending through the cancelllous part of C2 (Fig 8-6c)

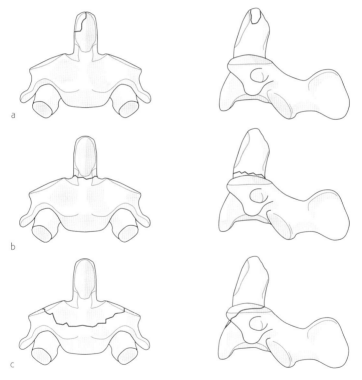

Fig 8-6a–c   Anderson classification of fractures of the odontoid process. Odontoid fracture AP and lateral view: a type I; b type II; c type III.

Treatment

Conservative treatment: A rigid neck collar or halo vest immobilization for all types.

Surgical treatment: Recommended for type II fractures of the odontoid process because of the tendency for pseudarthrosis formation. There are two surgical options: screw fixation of the odontoid or posterior fusion of C1/2.

■ Risk factor for pseudarthrosis: type II, >5 mm displacement, age >50 years, and posterior displacement.

Duration

Injury takes 3–4 months to heal.
Duration of disability is also 3–4 months.

Prognosis

Prognosis is good if there is no accompanying neurological deficit.

8.10   C3–C7 fracture (subaxial cervical spine injuries)

Mechanism of injury and types of injury

Motor vehicle injury, blunt trauma, or diving in shallow water.

Diagnostics

Physical examination: Neck pain and torticollis. Local injuries of the head and face at the site of the impact. Might have neurological injuries of the spinal cord and nerve roots.

X-ray examination: See algorithm on Fig 8-1.

Types of injury

I Flexion compression injury

■ Axial loading force, striking the back of the head. Diving into shallow water
■ Compression fracture of the vertebral body or fracture fragment of the anterior aspect of the vertebral body (teardrop fracture)

■ This fracture is unstable in flexion.

II Flexion distraction

■ Direct force, striking the occiput; subluxation or dislocation of facet joints

III Extension compression

- Direct force to the forehead and face, causing posterior displacement of the head, mainly in the elderly
- Fractures of the facet joints and pedicles with displacement of the vertebral body at the level of the fracture in relation to the inferior vertebral body. There is no kyphosis.

  - This injury is unstable in extension.

IV Extension distraction

- Direct force to the chin point, hanging. This injury is extremely rare. Diastasis at the level of the disc between vertebral bodies, usually with avulsion of the anterior aspect of the vertebral body (teardrop fracture)

  - This injury is universally unstable because of accompanying injury to the ligaments.

V Vertical compression (burst)

- Axial compression with fracture through the superior or inferior endplate

Treatment

Conservative treatment: Halo or cervical orthosis for stable fractures.

Surgical treatment: Reduction, spinal cord decompression, and fixation using an anterior and/or posterior approach.

The international Spine Trauma Study Group has developed the following algorithm (SLIC- Subaxial Injury Severity Score and Classification) for assessment of injury severity and the choice of treatment:

Morphology of injury

Compression	1 point
Burst	2 points
Distraction	3 points
Rotation/translation	4 points

Discoligamentary injury

Intact	0 points
Suspected	2 points
Disrupted	3 points

Neurological involvement

Intact	0 points
Root injury	1 point
Complete cord	2 points
Incomplete cord	3 points
Neuromodifier*	+1 point

* (continuous cord compression with neurodeficit)

Injury severity score is calculated by adding up the scores of each of the three items.
Treatment advice:
- 1–3 points: nonoperative
- 4 points: operative or nonoperative
- 5 points or more: operative

Duration
Injury takes 3–4 months to heal, depending on the type of fracture.
Duration of disability is 3–6 months.

Prognosis
Prognosis depends on the neurological injury and the levels involved. Some cervical spine function loss should be expected.

8.11 Fractures of spinous process or transverse process of cervical spine

Mechanism of injury
Direct force from impact of a blow or heavy object to the neck. Fatigue fracture of the C7 spinous process may occur in heavy manual laborers.

Clinical presentation
Neck pain with torticollis.

Diagnostics
Physical examination: Hypertonic musculature and torticollis. Local pain on palpation.
X-ray examination: X-rays of the cervical spine in two planes.

Classification
None.

Treatment
Conservative treatment: Analgesics and mobilization guided by the pain.
Surgical treatment: None.

Duration
Fracture takes 2–6 weeks to heal.
Duration of disability is 4 weeks.

Prognosis
Prognosis is good.

8.12   Fractures of the thoracolumbar spine

Mechanism of injury
High-energy injuries caused by falls from height or motor vehicle injury. Often seen in suicide attempts, too. Can also be seen with low-energy trauma in osteoporotic spine.

Clinical presentation
Back pain, sometimes associated with neurological deficit in the legs, grading according to the ASIA scale (Table 8-1).

Diagnostics
Preliminary examination: Any victim with high-energy trauma has spinal injury until proven otherwise. After stabilization of the vital parameters use the algorithm shown on Fig 8-7 for the imaging of the TL spine.

■ 80% of fractures occur between T10 and L2; imaging of the thoracolumbar junction should always be a priority.

Pending diagnosis: The patient should be lifted and turned by four people (head, thorax, pelvis, and legs).
Neurological examination: As soon as possible, including rectal examination and testing for sacral sensation.

Classification

Comprehensive classification (Magerl AO Classification of Thoracolumbar Fractures) is based on the model of a crane. There are three basic types (Fig 8-8):

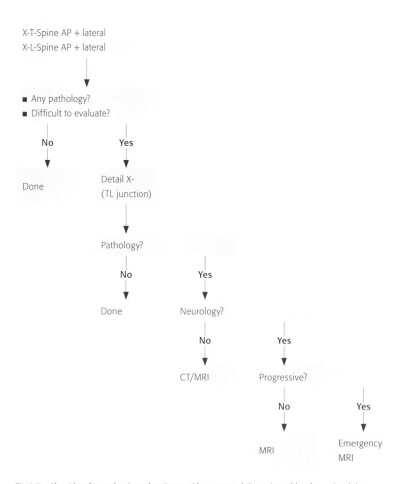

X-T-Spine AP + lateral
X-L-Spine AP + lateral

- Any pathology?
- Difficult to evaluate?

No → Done

Yes → Detail X- (TL junction)

Pathology?

No → Done

Yes → Neurology?

No → CT/MRI

Yes → Progressive?

No → MRI

Yes → Emergency MRI

Fig 8-7 Algorithm for evaluation of patients with suspected thoracic and lumbar spine injury.

Type A: Injury to the anterior elements (vertebral body and the disk) predominantly by compression forces. The posterior tension band is intact. Subclassification:

- A1: wedge-compression of the endplate
- A2: split fracture of the vertebral body
- A3: burst fracture

Type B: In addition to injury to the anterior elements there is also failure of the posterior tension band. Subclassification:

- B1: ligamentary failure of the tension band
- B2: osseous failure of the tension band
- B3: hyperextension injury

Type C: Anterior and posterior element injury with rotation. Subclassification:

- C1: type A injuries with rotation
- C2: type B injuries with rotation
- C3: rotational shear injuries

Injury Severity Score (TLICS): Spine Trauma Study Group has developed an injury severity and classification system. The following items are evaluated:

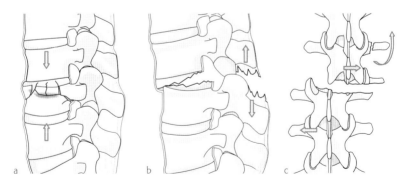

Fig 8-8a–c   Magerl AO Classification of Thoracolumbar Fractures: a type A—vertebral body compression; b type B—anterior and posterior element injury with distraction; c type C—anterior and posterior element injury with rotation.

Morphology:

Compression	1 point
Burst	2 points
Rotation/translation	3 points
Distraction	4 points

PLC (posterior ligamentary complex = tension band)

Intact	0 points
Suspected	2 points
Disrupted	3 points

Neurology

Intact	0 points
Root	2 points
Spinal cord/conus	
■ Complete	2 points
■ Incomplete	3 points
Cauda equina	3 points

The sum of the points from each of these three items makes the total TLICS score.

Treatment

The treatment algorithm proposed:

- TLICS score 1–3: conservative
- TLICS score 4: operative or conservative
- TLICS score 5 or more: operative

Clinical modifiers such as polytrauma, ankylosis of the spine, or the degree of deformity may add up to the basic TLICS score in the decision for conservative or operative treatment.

Conservative treatment: For compression fractures is functional—supportive or a brace for a short period (2–3 weeks) for pain relief. For burst fractures without neurology or PLC injury 8–12 weeks corset or orthosis.

Surgical treatment: Depending on the type and the surgical experience; anterior, posterior, or combined surgery.

- All patients older than 50 years with TL fractures should be screened for osteoporosis.

X-ray landmarks

AP view
1. Posterior rim (posterior wall)
2. Anterior rim (anterior wall)
3. Roof (superior articular surface)
4. Teardrop (relationship of columns)
6. Iliopectineal line (anterior column)
5. Ilioischial line (posterior column)

Iliac oblique view
1. Anterior rim (anterior wall)
2. Greater and lesser sciatic notch (posterior column)

Obturator oblique view
1. Posterior rim (posterior wall)
2. Pelvic brim (anterior column)

A CT scan of the pelvis can help in understanding the displacement of the fragments, presence of intraarticular fragment, femoral head injury, and size and impaction of the acetabular rim fracture.

A three-dimensional CT scan is not essential for treatment but gives a complete insight into the exact course of fracture lines.

Classification

The Letournel classification is based on the anatomy of the acetabulum and distinguishes five elementary and five complex types.

Elementary fractures	**Complex fractures**
Posterior wall	Posterior column + wall
Posterior column	Transverse + posterior wall
Anterior wall	T-shape
Anterior column	Anterior column + posterior hemitransverse
Transverse	Both columns

The most common fracture types are:
- Posterior wall
- Posterior column
- Anterior column
- Transverse and posterior wall
- T-shape

- Both columns
- Anterior column with posterior hemitransverse fracture

  ■ Central dislocation of hip, the commonly used term, should be avoided because medial dislocation of the femoral head can occur in many types of fractures.

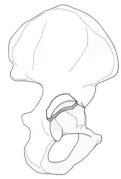

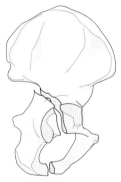

Fig 8-13   Fracture of the posterior wall of the acetabulum.

Fig 8-14   Fracture of the posterior column of the acetabulum.

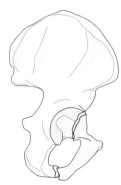

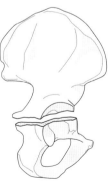

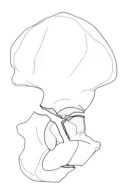

Fig 8-15   Fracture of the anterior column of the acetabulum.

Fig 8-16   Transverse fracture of the acetabulum.

Fig 8-17   T-shaped fracture of the acetabulum.

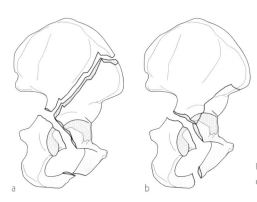

Fig 8-18a–b   Fracture of both columns of the acetabulum.

a

b

Treatment
Conservative treatment:
- Nondisplaced fractures
- With local infection or debridement of soft tissues
- In severe osteoporosis
- Fractures of both columns with secondary congruity
- Fractures of the lower anterior column and low transverse fractures
- Posterior wall fractures of less than 1/3 (in comparison with the unaffected side) of the width as measured on CT scan

Surgical treatment: Used for all fractures with displacement > 3 mm.

- Surgical treatment requires careful planning and a sound knowledge of the anatomy; extensive experience is needed to manage these fractures.

- Even with experts, it is only possible to obtain a good anatomical reconstruction in 75% of cases.

- Conservative treatment is the only correct choice in 10% of these fractures.

- Traction is not useful because a permanent reduction is not achieved and is not necessary in stable fractures. Pin-site problems caused by skeletal traction are common and can hinder surgical treatment. Skeletal traction with a pin inserted into the greater trochanter is no longer used.

Duration

Injury takes 6 weeks to heal.
Duration of disability is 3–4 months.

Prognosis

If conservative treatment is used as indicated, prognosis is good in 90% of cases and for surgical treatment in 75% of cases.

8.16 Hip dislocation

Mechanism of injury

High-energy trauma via the knee with the leg flexed and adducted (dashboard injury).

Clinical presentation

Leg in flexion, adduction, and internal rotation with posterior dislocation (95% of cases). Leg in extension, abduction, and external rotation with an anterior dislocation (5% of cases).

- Abdominal, chest, and head are commonly related injuries.

Diagnostics

Physical examination: Look for the characteristic position of the lower limb when dislocated. Palpation of the lower extremity searching for associated injuries, with particular attention to the knee joint. Neurological examination for sciatic nerve deficit.

X-ray examination: AP view of the pelvis. With posterior dislocation, the displaced femoral head is closer to the x-ray plate and thus appears smaller.

After reduction all views of the pelvis should be provided: inlet, outlet, obturator oblique, and iliac oblique views. Reduction should be concentric and joint space similar to the other side. It is also possible to evaluate associated fractures of the pelvis and acetabulum.

A CT scan is more sensitive to diagnose the joint congruence, intraarticular fragment, acetabular rim impaction, and femoral head fracture.

Classification
Posterior dislocation
Thompson Epstein classification:

Type I: pure dislocation or small posterior rim fracture
Type II: large posterior fragment
Type III: comminution of the posterior fragment
Type IV: associated acetabular fracture
Type V: associated femoral head fracture

Anterior dislocation
- Superior (pubic or subspinous)
- Inferior (obturator, thyroid, or perineal)

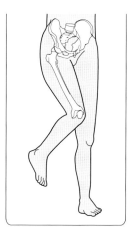 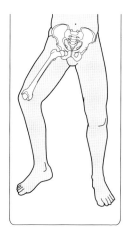

Fig 8-19   Hip dislocation with posterior displacement.

Fig 8-20   Hip dislocation with anterior displacement.

Treatment
Conservative treatment: Reduction as soon as possible with the patient under anesthesia, with muscle relaxation by traction to the leg with the hip in flexion and knee bent. Risks associated with reduction are damage to the sciatic nerve (keep the knee well bent), femoral head fracture (good muscle relaxation), and intraarticular displacement of the head and lip fragments. After reduction, stability is tested clinically and then an AP view is taken of the pelvis to assess the congruity of the joint. With CT scanning, fractures of

the posterior wall of the acetabulum, intraarticular fragments, or femoral head fractures can be evaluated.

Surgical treatment: For dislocation that cannot be reduced and redislocation after reduction. If, after reduction, CT scan shows a fracture of the posterior wall of the acetabulum of more than 1/3 (compared with the unaffected side), this should be fixed surgically.

Follow-up treatment: Mobilization can be started at once if the joint is stable after reduction. The joint is protected by letting the patient use crutches for ambulation for 3 weeks.

Duration
Injury lasts 3 weeks without a fracture; 6 weeks with a fracture.
Duration of disability is 6–12 weeks.

Prognosis
After early reduction, avascular necrosis of the femoral head occurs in less than 10% of cases.

8.17   Femoral head fracture

Mechanism of injury
Most commonly, motor vehicle high-energy trauma via the knee with the high flexed and adducted (dashboard injury).

Clinical presentation
The femoral head fracture is associated with hip dislocation, so in the posterior dislocated hip the lower limb will be shortened, adducted, and internally rotated.

Diagnostics
Physical examination: Look for the characteristic position of the lower limb when dislocated. Palpation of the lower extremity searching for associated injuries, with special attention to the knee joint. Neurological examination for sciatic nerve deficit.

X-ray examination: It is difficult to diagnose a femoral head fracture on AP views of the pelvis; a pelvic inlet view provides more information. A CT scan is indispensable.

Classification

Pipkin distinguishes four types:

Type 1:   hip dislocation with fracture of the femoral head inferior to the fovea capitus femoris

Type 2:   hip dislocation with fracture of the femoral head superior to the fovea capitus femoris, the fragment is joined to the teres ligament

Type 3:   type 1 or 2 injury associated with a fracture of the femoral neck

Type 4:   type 1 or 2 injury associated with a fracture of the acetabulum

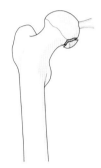

Fig 8-21   Fracture of the femoral head, Pipkin type 1.

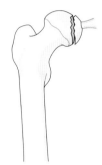

Fig 8-22   Fracture of the femoral head, Pipkin type 2.

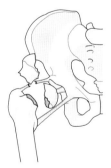

Fig 8-23   Fracture of the femoral head, Pipkin type 3.

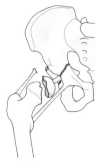

Fig 8-24   Fracture of the femoral head, Pipkin type 4.

Treatment
Conservative treatment: For types 1, 2, and 4 use closed reduction performed carefully because of the risk of a column fracture. If the fragment is not displaced, as seen on CT scan: 4 weeks traction in slight flexion.
Surgical treatment: For types 1, 2, and 4 if the fragment is displaced, remove if the fragment is small, and fix with screws if the fragment is large. For type 3: open reduction and fixation of both the femoral neck fracture and the femoral head fracture. In elderly patients, treatment consists of inserting head-neck prosthesis.

Duration
Injury takes 6 weeks to heal.
Duration of disability is 3–4 months.

Prognosis
Prognosis is generally worse than with a true hip dislocation because of the increased risk of femoral head necrosis and/or arthrosis.
After early reduction, avascular femoral head necrosis occurs in less than 10% of cases.

- Garden classification: There are four types based on the femoral head trabeculation pattern. Type I is a valgus-impacted fracture. It can be in slight retroversion or in neutral position. Type II is a complete fracture but undisplaced. There is no shift in alignment. Types III and IV are completely displaced fractures. Type III shows varus displacement and the trabecular line between femoral head and acetabulum forms an angle. Type IV shows complete separation of femoral head from the neck and the trabecular lines of femoral head and acetabulum realign.
- Müller AO Classification: 31-B1 is a subcapital fracture with slight displacement; 31-B2, a transcervical fracture; and 31-B3, a displaced nonimpacted fracture.

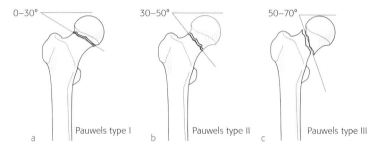

0–30°   30–50°   50–70°

a   Pauwels type I   b   Pauwels type II   c   Pauwels type III

Fig 9-1a–c   Pauwels classification of femoral neck fractures.

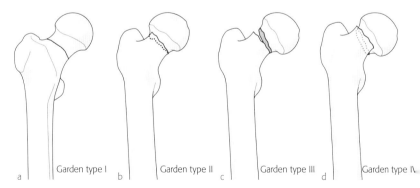

a   Garden type I   b   Garden type II   c   Garden type III   d   Garden type IV

Fig 9-2a–d   Garden classification of femoral neck fractures. a Garden type I, incomplete fracture; b Garden type II, complete fracture undisplaced; c Garden type III, complete displaced fracture with some bone contact; and d Garden type IV, complete displaced fracture with no bone contact.

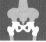

Treatment

Conservative treatment: This is reserved for stable fractures (Garden types I and II) in surgically unfit patients. With displacement, osteosynthesis should be done in patients younger than 65 years; otherwise prosthesis should be considered in patients older than 65 years.

Surgical treatment: For displaced or unstable fractures (Garden types II, III, and IV): osteosynthesis in patients younger than 65 years. Closed or open reduction on the extension table. Osteosynthesis with screws or plate-sliding screw devices (DHS). Use head-neck prosthesis in older patients or total hip replacement depending on the patients' physiological age and their functional requirements. In children: gentle reduction and pins or screws osteosynthesis as soon as possible if the fracture is displaced. Postoperatively, the hip can be immobilized in spica cast.

Follow-up treatment: Up to 8 weeks (partial) weight-bearing mobilization.

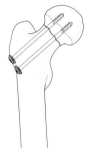

Fig 9-3   Femoral neck fracture treated with screws.

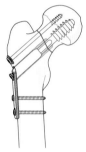

Fig 9-4   Femoral neck fracture treated with plate-sliding screw device.

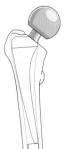

Fig 9-5   Femoral neck fracture treated with head-neck (hemi-)prosthesis.

Duration

Fracture takes 8–12 weeks to heal.
Duration of disability is 12–16 weeks.

Prognosis

Mortality after hip fractures ranges from 14–50% in the first year depending largely on the patient's comorbidities. After osteosynthesis, pseudarthrosis or nonunion occurs in 10–30% of cases; avascular necrosis of the femoral head, 10–45%. The incidence increases according to the initial displacement and is also related to the accuracy of reduction. After head-neck prosthesis: reoperation in 5–10% of patients because of dislocation, protrusion, periprosthetic fracture, or loosening of prosthesis.

9.2   Pertrochanteric femoral fractures

Mechanism of injury

Direct force caused by a fall on the trochanteric area. Fractures in younger people are usually due to high-energy trauma, like motor vehicle injuries or fall from height. In the elderly, most of these fractures are caused by a simple fall and are low energy.

Clinical presentation

Lower extremity shortened and externally rotated, pain, and loss of function.

Diagnostics

Physical examination: Shortening and external rotation of the lower extremity, depending on the displacement. Loss of function.

X-ray examination: AP view of the pelvis and lateral view of the hip. The fracture line extends through or between the greater and lesser trochanter, sometimes crossing the subtrochanteric area.

Classification

The essence of both Evans-Johnson and Müller AO Classification is the differentiation between stable and unstable (comminuted) fractures.
Evans-Johnson classification: types 1 and 2, stable; types 3–5, unstable.
Müller AO Classification: 31-A1, 31-A2.1, 31-A2.2, stable; 31-A2.3, 31-A3, unstable.

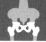
Treatment

Conservative treatment: Skeletal traction for 8–10 weeks is technically possible but not acceptable socially, economically, or medically (in the elderly). It is rarely used today. It requires meticulous nursing care with emphasis on prevention of pressure sores, hypostatic pneumonia, and poor nutrition. Patients who survive have a short, externally rotated leg and are unlikely ever to walk again.

Surgical treatment: For stable fractures, osteosynthesis by using a plate-sliding screw device (DHS). For unstable fractures, osteosynthesis by using cephalomedullary devices (Gamma nail or PFNA) or using fixed angled devices (angled blade plate or DCS). Closed reduction is achieved on a traction table. After fixation, most patients should be allowed weight-bearing walking.

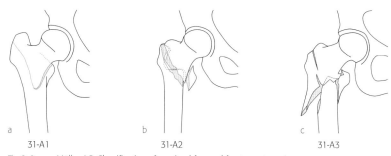

a   31-A1   b   31-A2   c   31-A3

Fig 9-6a–c   Müller AO Classification of proximal femoral fractures, type A.

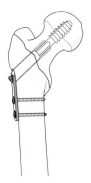

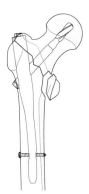

Fig 9-7   Stable pertrochanteric femoral fracture treated with plate-sliding screw device (DHS).

Fig 9-8   Unstable pertrochanteric femoral fracture treated with cephalomedullary device.

Duration
Fracture takes 6–8 weeks to heal.
Duration of disability is 3–4 months depending mostly on patients' comorbidities.

Prognosis
After appropriate osteosynthesis, prognosis is favorable. A minimal loss of hip mobility is present.

9.3   Subtrochanteric fractures

Mechanism of injury
Direct or axial force with or without torsion in young patients (high energy). In older people, severe osteoporosis or pathological fractures may result in subtrochanteric fractures with low energy.

Clinical presentation
Lower extremity shortened, externally rotated, and painful.

Diagnostics
Physical examination: Swelling, loss of function, and obvious displacement of the lower extremity.
X-ray examination: X-rays of the hip and the entire femur in two planes. The fracture line is below the level of the lesser trochanter.

- Consider tumor (metastasis) as a cause of pathological fracture.

Classification
Müller AO Classification: 32-A(1–3).1, 32-B(1–3).1, 32-C(1–3).1.
Russel-Taylor classification: type I, no piriformis fossa extension; type II, with piriformis fossa extension (involves greater trochanter).

Treatment
Conservative treatment: In children aged 0–3 years, Bryant traction for 3 weeks in clinic or at home (Fig 9-10) followed by a pelvis-leg plaster cast for 1–3 weeks. In children aged 4–10 years, 90/90 traction according to Weber (Fig 9-11); if good position is achieved after 4–6 weeks (in clinic or at home), then pelvis-leg (weight-bearing) plaster cast for 2–6 weeks.

Surgical treatment: Nearly all subtrochanteric fractures are unstable fractures, osteosynthesis is best achieved by dynamic condylar screw (DCS), 95° angled blade plate, trochanteric stabilization plate, or a cephalomedullary device (Gamma nail or PFNA). Reduction is difficult in displaced fractures because the glutei and psoas attached to the proximal fragment, pull it into flexion and abduction while the adductors attached to this distal fragment pull it into adduction. Frequently an open reduction is required.

Follow-up treatment: For adequately fixed fractures, patients could usually be allowed to start certain degree of weight-bearing walking exercise.

Duration

Fracture takes 8–10 weeks to heal.
Duration of disability is 3–4 months.

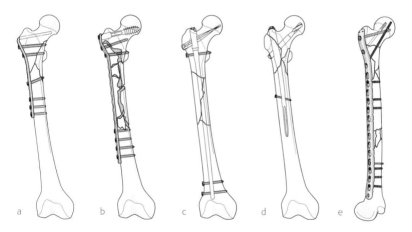

Fig 9-9a–e   Five options for stabilizing subtrochanteric fractures.

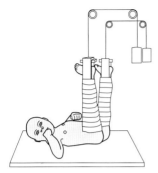

Fig 9-10   Treatment of a subtrochanteric fracture of the femoral shaft in an infant according to Bryant.

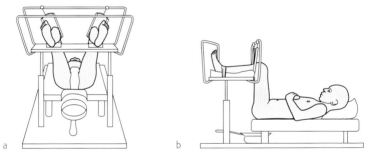

a   b

Fig 9-11a–b   Treatment of a subtrochanteric fracture of the femoral shaft in a child according to Weber.

Prognosis

The prognosis is good, provided the right implant is used and a good reduction is obtained.

9.4   Fractures of the femoral shaft

Mechanism of injury
Direct and/or axial force. In younger patients, almost always the result of high-energy trauma, for example, motor vehicle injury, pedestrian hit by a vehicle, or fall from height. For older patients, these fractures could be caused by a simple fall in combination with osteoporosis (low energy).

Clinical presentation
Swelling, deformity, loss of function, and pain are usual symptoms. For high-energy trauma, it is frequently associated with other injuries of the musculoskeletal system; for example, ipsilateral femoral neck fractures, intertrochanteric fractures, or injuries to other body systems such as a head or chest injury (polytrauma).

Diagnostics
Physical examination: Characteristic clinical picture including swelling and obvious external rotation. The hemodynamic status should be monitored because femoral shaft fractures can result in substantial blood loss hematoma. The examination of the spine, pelvis, and adjacent joints is important to exclude associated injuries especially in young patients with high-energy trauma.
X-ray examination: X-rays of the upper leg in two planes including the hip and knee joint.

> ■ Also consider ipsilateral pelvic fracture, hip dislocation, or proximal femoral fracture. The hip cannot be examined clinically, so an x-ray of the pelvis should always be taken.

Classification
Shaft fractures are classified according to site of injury, degree of displacement, fracture anatomy (simple or multiple), and according to severity of the injury of the soft tissue—both open and closed.
Müller AO Classification: 32-A, 32-B, 32-C (Fig 9-12).

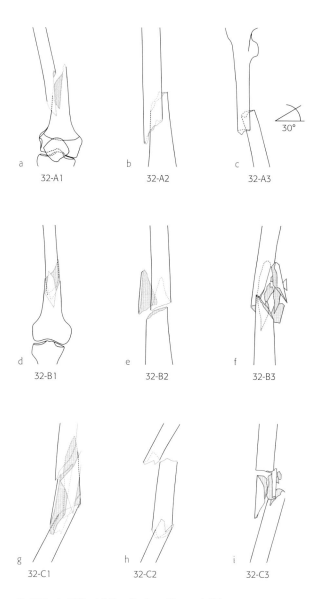

a 32-A1

b 32-A2

c 30° 32-A3

d 32-B1

e 32-B2

f 32-B3

g 32-C1

h 32-C2

i 32-C3

Fig 9-12a–i Müller AO Classification of femur shaft fractures.

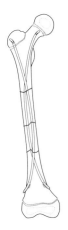

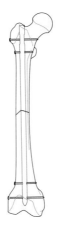

Fig 9-13   Femoral shaft fracture in a child treated by intramedullary pins.

Fig 9-14   Femoral shaft fracture in an adult treated by an intramedullary locking nail.

Treatment

Conservative treatment: In children aged 0–3 years used longitudinal or Gallows traction for 3 weeks (in the clinic or at home), followed by a pelvis-leg plaster cast for 3 weeks. In children aged 3–5 years, 90/90 traction according to Weber (in the clinic or at home) for 4–6 weeks, then pelvis-leg plaster for 4–6 weeks.

- In children, the aim should be consolidation with some shortening (not more than 2 cm) because of compensatory growth.

Surgical treatment: In children 3–10 years, intramedullary fixation (Prevot, Nancy, Rush) (Fig 9-13). In children aged 10–16, osteosynthesis with plate or intramedullary pin. In adults, osteosynthesis or intramedullary (locking) nail (Fig 9-14). Reamed nailing is usually considered to be better than unreamed nailing with respect to union rate. However, the consideration should be based on the individual situation, eg, open fracture, multiple-injured unstable patients. An alternative is plate osteosynthesis, especially in the presence of hip and knee prostheses. Locking plate fixation using minimally invasive technique is another option in special situations, eg, extremely narrow intramedullary canal, irregular shape of the femur, and so on.

- Be aware of rotation errors with intramedullary fixation.

Duration

In children, fracture takes 3–8 weeks to heal, depending on the age; in adults 8–12 weeks.

Duration of disability is 4 months.

Prognosis

Prognosis is good, provided length, axis, and rotation are correct.

9.5   Supracondylar fractures of the femur (extraarticular)

Mechanism of injury

In young adults, it is usually due to an axial force with a varus, valgus, or rotational force as the result of high-energy trauma, eg, motor vehicle injury or fall from height. It can also happen in older patients with osteoporotic bone after a simple fall. A particular group of patients is those bed-bound or chair-bound with contracted knees. A supracondylar fracture may occur with forceful movement of the involved limb during transfer (low energy).

Clinical presentation

Swelling, deformity, loss of function, and pain. Open wound is not rare in high-energy trauma.

Diagnostics

Physical examination: A typical clinical picture is swollen knee area, obvious displacement of the bone. Distal neurovascular status should be checked in all injuries.

X-ray examination: X-rays in two planes of the entire femur (including hip) and good x-rays of the knee. Gentle traction film may help in better delineation of fracture pattern.

- In children, differentiate from epiphysiolysis.

Classification

This is an extraarticular fracture that is classified according to the degree of displacement, single and multiple and comminutive, open or closed, and according to the severity of the soft-tissue injury.

Müller AO Classification: 33-A(1–3).

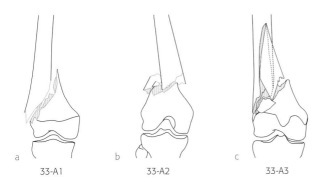

a   33-A1   b   33-A2   c   33-A3

Fig 9-15a–c   Müller AO Classification of distal femur fractures, type A (extraarticular fractures).

Treatment
Conservative treatment: In children (often a nondisplaced or greenstick fracture), plaster cast to the upper leg for 4–6 weeks.
Surgical treatment: Osteosynthesis with 95° angled blade plate (Fig 9-16) or dynamic condylar screw (DCS). For simple fracture configuration, open reduction with anatomical reduction is the choice of treatment. For comminuted fracture, close reduction and internal fixation using minimally invasive technique is the better choice of treatment. The implant can be a dynamic condylar screw, less invasive stabilization system (LISS) plate (Fig 9-17), or supracondylar retrograde nail. The LISS can be particularly helpful in osteoporotic bone.
In children with a displaced fracture: closed repositioning and fixation with crossed K-wires, followed by upper leg plaster cast for 6 weeks (Fig 9-18).

Duration
Fracture takes 3–6 months to heal depending on the mode of stabilization. Duration of disability is about 6–9 months. The length of rehabilitation also depends on the associated soft-tissue injury.

Prognosis
Prognosis is good; some limitation to knee extension may remain due to adhesions in the extension apparatus.

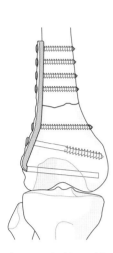

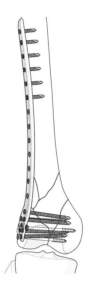

Fig 9-16   Distal femoral fracture treated with 95° angled blade plate and screws.

Fig 9-17   Distal femoral fracture treated with LISS.

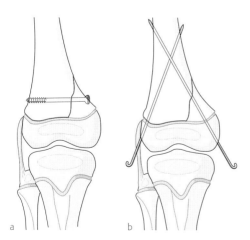

Fig 9-18a–b   Distal femoral fracture in a child treated with: a screw fixation; b K-wire fixation.

9.6   Injuries of the metaphysis of the distal femur

Mechanism of injury
In Salter-Harris types I and II injuries and avulsion fractures of the collateral lateral ligament, indirect force resulting in varus or valgus deformity or hyperextension injury. In Salter-Harris types III and IV injuries: mainly indirect axial force (see chapter 3: Principles of fracture treatment).

- In children the ligaments are stronger than the metaphysis.

Clinical presentation
Hemarthrosis in types III and IV. Type V presents as an injury to the ligament. Types I and II can result in severe gait abnormalities.

Diagnostics
Physical examination: Swelling, deformity, loss of function (hemarthrosis).

- Due to the minimal abnormality in type V injuries, the correct diagnosis is easily missed.

X-ray examination: X-rays in two planes of the entire femur (including hip) and good x-rays of the knee. CT scans and MRI are helpful in evaluating occult fractures.

- Epiphysiolysis that is not or only slightly displaced can be shown by varus and valgus stress x-rays.

Classification
According to Salter-Harris (see chapter 3: Principles of fracture treatment):
Type I: Fracture through zone of ossification
Type II: Fracture through zone of ossification with metaphyseal fragment
Type III: Epiphyseal fracture
Type IV: Epiphyseal fracture extending to the metaphysis (Fig 9-19)
Type V: Compression of the growth plate

Treatment

Conservative treatment: Types I and II, if stable after repositioning use long plaster cast for 6–8 weeks, depending on age.

- Most type II injuries are unstable and will slip if internal fixation is not used.

Surgical treatment: Unstable types I and II, repositioning and crossed K-wires or screw osteosynthesis (type II). To prevent growth disorders: anatomical repositioning and screw fixation in types III, IV, and V.

Follow-up treatment: In cases of unstable osteosynthesis on exercise, additional immobilization (plaster cast) for 4–8 weeks may be needed.

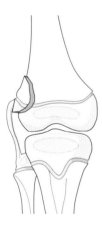

Fig 9-19   Salter-Harris type IV epiphysiolysis.

Duration

Fracture takes 6–8 weeks to heal.

Prognosis

There is a risk of premature closure of the metaphysis, especially in types III, IV, and V injuries. Anatomical repositioning reduces this risk considerably. The distal epiphysis contributes the most to the growth of the upper leg (70%). Growth disorders are therefore severe. Corrective surgery, such as lengthening (in case of shortening) and osteotomy (in case of axial defects), is sometimes necessary during the growing period.

10 Knee and lower leg injuries

10   Knee and lower leg injuries

10.1   Intraarticular fractures of the distal femur

Mechanism of injury
Direct high-energy force from a motor vehicle collision or fall from height. Depending on the position of the lower extremity at the time of impact, the medial, lateral, or both condyles may be involved. Müller AO Classification 33-B(1–3), and 33-C(1–3) (Fig 10-1).

Clinical presentation
Pain in the lower thigh and knee, swelling and deformity around the knee joint; weight bearing is not possible.

Diagnostics
Physical examination: Hemarthrosis with a nearly normal contour of the patella and the extensor mechanism. Obvious deformity. Passive movements of the knee are painful.

- Check for accompanying vascular injuries.

- In a child with hemarthrosis, always consider the possibility of an injury to the growth zone.

X-ray examination: X-rays of the knee in two planes, with oblique views if necessary. A computed tomographic (CT) scan is useful for delineating intraarticular fracture lines and preoperative planning.

Classification
- Monocondylar fracture of the lateral or medial femoral condyle (saggital fracture): Müller AO Classification 33-B(1–2)
- Monocondylar fracture of the posterior condyle (coronal fracture): Müller AO Classification 33-B3
- T- or Y-fractures: Müller AO Classification 33-C(1–3)

Accompanying injuries to the ligaments or menisci occur less commonly with fractures of the distal femur than with fractures of the tibial plateau.

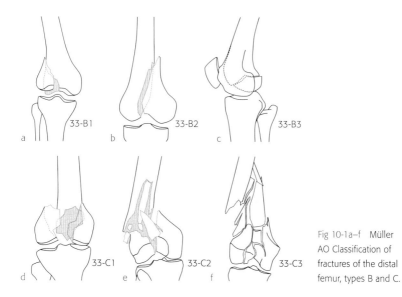

Fig 10-1a–f Müller AO Classification of fractures of the distal femur, types B and C.

Treatment

Conservative treatment: Rarely indicated and is reserved for nonambulatory patients with minimal to mild displacement or for patients too sick for surgery. A hinged knee brace is adequate stabilization for this group of patients.

Surgical treatment: Nearly always indicated; osteosynthesis with screws, 95° angled blade plate, and 95° dynamic condylar screw (DCS), locking plate, or retrograde intramedullary nail.

Follow-up treatment: After osteosynthesis, start exercises straight away using an elastic bandage or a continuous passive motion (CPM) device at first, if necessary. Next, start active exercises and partial weight bearing on crutches when there is evidence of healing (8–12 weeks).

Duration

Injury takes 8–12 weeks to heal.
Duration of disability is 3–6 months.

Prognosis

Prognosis is good if anatomical position is achieved. There is a high risk of arthrosis with a nonanatomical position.

10.2   Quadriceps tendon rupture

Mechanism of injury
Indirect trauma, forced contraction of the quadriceps muscles with flexed knee. Often in combination with a systemic disease, such as rheumatoid arthritis, uremia, and/or long-term use of corticosteroids (in patients > 50 years).

Clinical presentation
Hemarthrosis. With a complete rupture, inability to actively extend the knee or lift the leg while in extension.

Diagnostics
Physical examination: Palpable defect directly proximal to the patella.
X-ray examination: X-rays of the knee in two planes show inferior displacement of the patella, sometimes associated with avulsion fragments of the superior pole. Ultrasound or MRI is invaluable in cases of partial rupture.

Classification
None.

Treatment
Conservative treatment: In small incomplete ruptures use walking cast with the knee in extension for 6 weeks, quadriceps-strengthening exercises.
Surgical treatment: For complete or more than 50% partial ruptures use fixation of the tendon on the patella through drill holes or with anchors in the superior pole of the patella (Fig 10-2).
Follow-up treatment: Walking cast or knee brace with the knee in extension for 6 weeks, quadriceps-strengthening exercises.

Duration
Injury takes 6 weeks to heal.
Duration of disability is 3–12 months.

Prognosis
Prognosis is good. A 5–10° restriction in active knee extension can persist because of lengthening of the tendon or adhesions of muscles.

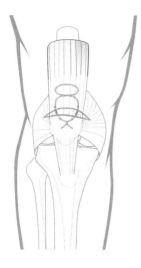

Fig 10-2 Treatment of the quadriceps tendon with sutures through drill holes in the superior pole of the patella.

10.3 Patella fractures

Mechanism of injury
Indirect trauma from forced contraction of the quadriceps muscles because of a fall or from a direct blow or impact (dashboard).

Clinical presentation
Hemarthrosis, local contusion or abrasions of the skin, inability to actively extend the knee, or lift the leg in extension (when the extensor mechanism is damaged).

Diagnostics
Physical examination: Sometimes a palpable defect, the joint is swollen.
X-ray examination: X-rays of the knee in three planes, ie, AP, lateral, and tangential patella views (the last if pain permits).

Classification
- Extraarticular, partial articular vertical, complete articular transverse—comminuted fractures (Fig 10-3)
- According to the degree of displacement

■ May be associated with patella bipartita; if in doubt, take a comparative AP view of the other knee.

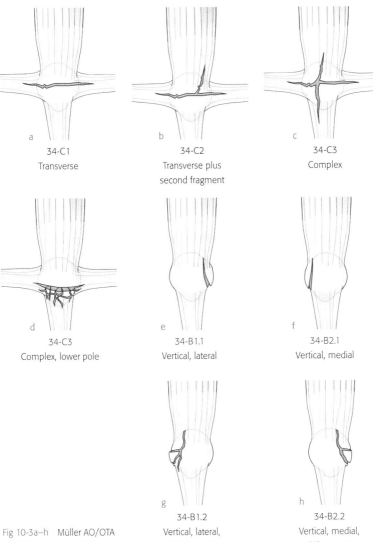

a
34-C1
Transverse

b
34-C2
Transverse plus
second fragment

c
34-C3
Complex

d
34-C3
Complex, lower pole

e
34-B1.1
Vertical, lateral

f
34-B2.1
Vertical, medial

g
34-B1.2
Vertical, lateral,
multifragmentary

h
34-B2.2
Vertical, medial,
multifragmentary

Fig 10-3a–h   Müller AO/OTA
Classification of patella fractures.

Treatment

Conservative treatment: In fractures with an intact extensor mechanism and minimal displacement (< 2 mm) use walking cast with the knee in slight flexion for 6 weeks, quadriceps-strengthening exercises.

Surgical treatment: In fractures with a wide fracture gap because of a damaged extensor mechanism or displacement (> 2 mm) use reconstruction, generally with tension band osteosynthesis (Fig 10-4), possibly in combination with screw fixation. In partial patellectomy: resection of the inferior pole is generally used with refixation of the patella tendon on the patella. In total patellectomy: suturing of the retinaculum and what is left of the tendon.

Follow-up treatment: With stable fixation, functional treatment is permitted with active flexion and extension, quadriceps-strengthening exercises, using a walking cast or brace if necessary for 6 weeks. With partial or total patellectomy: walking cast or brace with the knee in extension for 6 weeks, quadriceps-strengthening exercises.

Duration

In most cases injury takes 6 weeks to heal.
Duration of disability is 3–6 months.

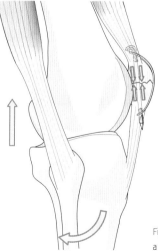

Fig 10-4   Transverse fracture of the patella treated with a tension band.

Prognosis

After successful osteosynthesis and partial patellectomy (mild) pain often persists and there is a risk of patellofemoral arthrosis. After total patellectomy, persisting pain is rare but a clear quadriceps dystrophy may remain with a corresponding weakness and/or extensor lag.

- Prognosis of late patellectomy is less favorable because of posttraumatic arthrosis of the knee.

10.4   Patella dislocation

Mechanism of injury

Indirect trauma caused by forced flexion of the knee with external rotation of the lower leg.

- Watch out for dysplasia of the patella or the lateral femoral condyle, sometimes associated with genu valgum.

Clinical presentation

Knee in flexion with springy elastic resistance, pronating medial femoral condyle; the patella is displaced laterally.

Diagnostics

Physical examination: Characteristic clinical picture if luxation is still present (see above). After (spontaneous) reduction: hemarthrosis, pain at the level of the medial retinaculum (Fig 10-5).

X-ray examination: X-rays of the knee in three planes, ie, AP, lateral, and tangential patella view.

- Look out for an osteochondral fracture of the medial patella facet or the lateral femoral condyle.

Classification

None.

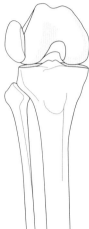

Fig 10-5   Dislocation of the patella (always laterally).

Treatment

Conservative treatment: Reduction after good pain management or under (regional) anesthesia; the knee is extended with local pressure to manipulate the patella medially. Next a cast or brace with the knee flexed to 10° for 4–6 weeks. Quadriceps-strengthening exercises.

Surgical treatment: Used in osteochondral fractures of the lateral femoral condyle or the patella joint area. Also used for repeated dislocation secondary to hypermobility of the patella.

Duration

Injury takes 6 weeks to heal.
Duration of disability is 8 weeks.

Prognosis

Prognosis is good; sometimes recurrent patella dislocation results which requires surgical treatment.

10.5 Patella tendon rupture

Mechanism of injury
Indirect trauma from forced contraction of the quadriceps muscles with the knee flexed. May occur as a complication of local steroid injection.

Clinical presentation
Hemarthrosis; inability to actively extend the knee and lift the leg when in extension.

Diagnostics
Physical examination: Palpable defect under the patella (Fig 10-6).
X-ray examination: X-rays of the knee in two planes. Superior displacement of the patella, sometimes with avulsion of the inferior pole.

Classification
None.

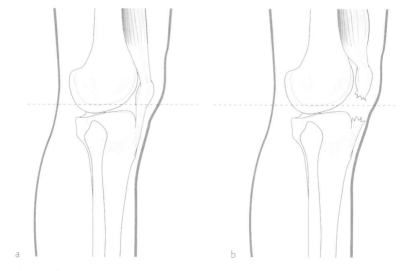

Fig 10-6a–b   a Normal position of the patella in relation to the knee joint. b Rupture of the patellar tendon with superior displacement of the patella in relation to the joint line.

Treatment

Conservative treatment: This injury almost always requires surgical repair.

Surgical treatment: Fixation of the tendon to the patella through drill holes or anchors in the inferior pole. To protect the reconstruction, a figure-of-eight cerclage wire can be attached around the patella and through the drill hole in the tibial tuberosity (Fig 10-7).

Follow-up treatment: A walking cast or knee brace with the knee in extension for 6 weeks, quadriceps-strengthening exercises.

Duration

Injury takes 6 weeks to heal.
Duration of disability is 3 months.

Prognosis

Prognosis is good but full flexion is rarely obtained.

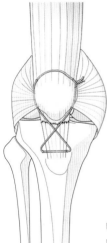

Fig 10-7   Rupture of the patellar tendon treated with sutures in combination with supporting tension band.

10.6 Medial collateral ligament rupture

Ruptures of the capsular ligament of the knee are nearly always combination injuries because multiple ligamentous structures are usually involved, while damage to the menisci and joint cartilage can also occur. Injuries of the different ligamentous structures are discussed separately because diagnostics and treatment also need to be looked at separately.

Mechanism of injury

Valgus of the knee is caused by direct or indirect trauma to the lateral aspect of the leg (Fig 10-8). An isolated injury of the medial ligament occurs if the force is moderate. The ligament can tear because of overextension. With greater impact, the injury not only affects the ligament but also damages the meniscus and/or the cruciate ligament ("unhappy triad").

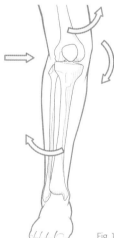

Fig 10-8   Mechanism injury of a rupture of the medial collateral ligament.

Clinical presentation

Pain and mild swelling of the medial aspect of the knee. Weight bearing is possible but usually the patient holds the knee in slight flexion.

Diagnostics

Physical examination: Swelling and pain on palpation of the medial aspect of the knee, either over the ligament or at the insertion to the medial condyle and/or proximal tibia. Hemarthrosis is usually minimal. The knee is stable in extension. On valgus stress in 30° flexion, medial laxity usually occurs.

- If the knee is unstable in extension, cruciate ligaments are also damaged.

X-ray examination: To exclude bone abnormalities and avulsions, standard x-rays of the knee in two planes are adequate.

Other examinations: Used if there is swelling of the joint—aspiration to ascertain if hemarthrosis is present. An MRI is useful if injury to the meniscus is suspected.

Classification

- Partial tear or strain of the medial collateral ligament
- Isolated tear of the medial ligament, without further abnormalities
- Ligamentous injury with damage to the meniscus and sometimes also to the cruciate ligaments

Treatment

Conservative treatment: In case of MCL strain use a hinged knee brace or immobilizing bandage, muscle training, and resting the knee for several weeks. With an isolated tear of the medial ligament use immobilization in a cast or brace for 4 weeks, then mobilize and extend the range of exercises.

Surgical treatment: When a tear of the medial ligament is related to other injuries.

- Definitive surgery to associated anterior cruciate ligament injuries may best be delayed until hemarthrosis is fully resolved.

Follow-up treatment: After surgery, 4–5 weeks in a cast or brace followed by a brace and exercises.

Duration

A strain injury takes 2–3 weeks to heal and a rupture 6 weeks.

Duration of disability is 3 weeks in minor injuries and 10–12 weeks for a complete rupture.

Prognosis

Prognosis is good if the anatomical proportions can be restored and the patient ensures good strength and function in thigh muscles. Chronic functional instability of the medial ligament is extremely rare, even if the abduction stress test remains positive.

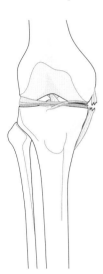

Fig 10-9   Rupture of the medial collateral ligament, with injury to the meniscus.

10.7   Lateral collateral ligament rupture

Mechanism of injury

Direct or indirect trauma to the medial aspect of the leg causing varus of the knee.

Clinical presentation

Pain on the external aspect of the knee, weight bearing is possible but painful.

Diagnostics

Physical examination: Swelling and pain on palpation of the external aspect of the knee. Hemarthrosis is usually minimal. The knee is stable in extension. On varus stress in 30° flexion, laxity usually occurs (Fig 10-10).

- With serious injury, assess for deficit of the peroneal nerve.

X-ray examination: X-rays of the knee in two planes to exclude bone abnormalities. Sometimes avulsion of the anterolateral margin of the tibia (deep lateral ligament) or of the fibular head (pull-off injury caused by superficial ligament or tendon of the biceps muscle) can occur. On suspicion of meniscus and/or other intraarticular injuries, MRI is indicated.

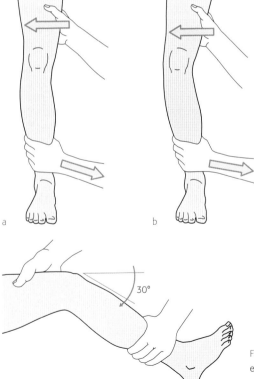

Fig 10-10a–c   The knee is examined in 30° flexion and a varus stress applied.

Classification

- Partial tear or strain of the fibular collateral ligament or avulsion fractures or the fibular head (Fig 10-11)
- Rupture of the ligament related to injury to the dorsolateral capsule, the meniscus, and/or cruciate ligaments

Treatment

Conservative treatment: With lateral collateral ligament strain use a hinged knee brace and/or pressure bandage and gradually increasing exercises with muscle training. With an isolated rupture, immobilization in a cast for 4–5 weeks, quadriceps-strengthening exercises.

Surgical treatment: For ruptures associated with meniscus injury and/or injury of the dorsolateral structures. The aim should be to obtain an accurate restoration of the anatomical proportions by ensuring the dorsolateral structures are at the correct tension.

Follow-up treatment: Postoperative cast or brace to protect lateral structures. After 4 weeks, gradually increasing exercises with focus on strengthening the musculature.

Duration

A strain injury takes 3 weeks to heal and complete rupture 6–8 weeks.
Duration of disability is 3 weeks to 3 months depending on the type of injury.

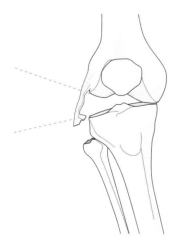

Fig 10-11 Avulsion fracture of the fibular head.

Prognosis

Prognosis is generally good if the anatomical proportions can be restored and the patient achieves good muscular strength.

■ Chronic posterolateral instability results in considerable functional restriction.

10.8 Anterior cruciate ligament rupture

Mechanism of injury

Usually indirect trauma to the medial or lateral aspect of the leg. The foot is often set on the ground and a valgus or varus rotation occurs. Another mechanism of injury is hyperextension of the knee. An injury to the anterior cruciate ligament is often linked with injuries to the medial or lateral collateral structures and often also the meniscus. Isolated injuries of the anterior cruciate ligaments are rare.

Clinical presentation

Acute pain, swelling of the knee. Moving and weight bearing are painful; with severe swelling the knee is held in flexion.

Diagnostics

Physical examination: Hemarthrosis is present. The drawer test is usually positive; ie, at 90° flexion of the knee the tibia can be moved anteriorly in relation to the femur (Fig 10-12). More reliable is the Lachman test: at 20−30° flexion of the knee, the tibia is moved anteriorly in relation to the femur. When the posterior cruciate ligament is intact, the Pivot shift can be positive; ie, anterolateral subluxation can be manipulated on internal rotation/valgus stress to the knee. If the patient has severe pain, the knee can only be examined adequately with he/she anesthetized.

X-ray examination: X-rays of the knee in two planes to exclude bone abnormalities. Avulsion of the tibial spines (ACL origin) can best be seen with a tunnel view. An avulsion of the lateral joint capsule from lateral rim of the tibial plateau (Segund sign) is also commonly seen with ACL injuries.

Other examinations: Aspiration of the joint to demonstrate hemarthrosis. If in doubt about the severity of the injury to the soft-tissue structures (the meniscus), an MRI is indicated.

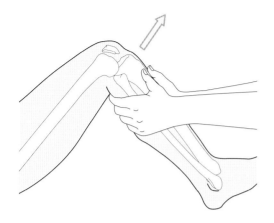

Fig 10-12   Applying the drawer test in ruptures of the cruciate ligament.

Classification
- Partial injury to the anterior cruciate ligament
- Avulsion of the insertion at the femur or the tibial plateau
- Complete mid-substance tear

Treatment
Conservative treatment: For partial cruciate ligament injuries and full interligamentous injuries if there is no accompanying damage to the menisci and/or the collateral ligaments. Treatment consists of exercises and muscle training. Do not immobilize in a cast or brace. Approximately 30–50% of patients do not have functional instability.

Surgical treatment: Direct suture repair of the anterior cruciate ligament is not helpful because a mid-substance tear does not heal. Boney avulsions are reinserted (Fig 10-13). Treatment of the accompanying injuries of both the meniscus and collateral ligaments of the capsular structures is needed for an optimal recovery of peripheral stability. In athletes, primary reconstruction/plasty of the anterior cruciate ligament should be considered.

Follow-up treatment: After reinsertion of an avulsion fracture use a hinged knee brace with the knee in slight flexion for 6 weeks followed by exercises. After suturing of the meniscus and peripheral structures, immobilization for 4–6 weeks is necessary followed by a brace treatment for 4 weeks. Exercises can gradually be started with focus on muscle strength.

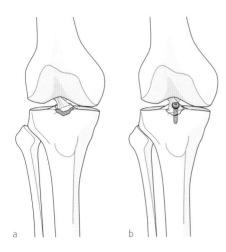

Fig 10-13a–b a Cruciate ligament injury with osseous avulsion; b fixation with screw.

Duration

Injury takes 6–10 weeks to heal, depending on the severity of the injury to other structures.

Duration of disability is 6 weeks to 12 months depending on professional activities.

Prognosis

Of patients with a complete rupture of the anterior cruciate ligament, 75% achieve good function when the muscular stability has recovered; the rest need secondary reconstruction of the anterior cruciate ligament.

10.9   Posterior cruciate ligament rupture

Mechanism of injury

Direct force to the tibia while the knee is flexed from a fall or a motor vehicle collision (dashboard injury). Hyperextension of the knee.

Clinical presentation

Pain in the knee, and swelling of the knee or the popliteal space. Knee pain on joint loading.

■ This injury is sometimes associated with a fracture of the patella, femoral shaft, acetabulum, or posterior hip dislocation.

Diagnostics

Physical examination: With the knee flexed, the lower leg is displaced posteriorly in relation to the thigh. Both legs should be compared at 90° flexion in hips and knees (Fig 10-14). The posterior drawer test is positive with the knee flexed to 90°; this injury is often also associated with posterolateral instability.

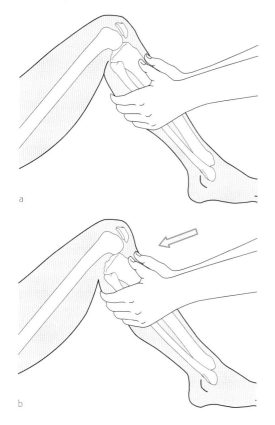

Fig 10-14a–b   a Knee in posterior drawer position; b test is positive.

■ It is difficult to differentiate between the anterior and posterior drawer phenomenon. With a rupture of the posterior cruciate ligament, the Lachman test is negative.

X-ray examination: X-rays of the knee in two planes to exclude bone injuries. Injury to the posterior cruciate ligament is often associated with an avulsion of the boney insertion into the proximal tibia.

Other examinations: Aspiration of the knee if hemarthrosis is present. MRI is indicated when other injuries, such as damage to the meniscus, are suspected.

Classification
■ Strain injury
■ Avulsion fracture of the insertion of the posterior cruciate ligament into the proximal tibia
■ Mid-substance tears
■ Injury of the posterior cruciate ligament combined with other lesions

Treatment
Conservative treatment: With strain injuries and slight instability use pressure bandage, muscle training exercises.
Surgical treatment: For avulsion fractures, in case of severe instability due to ligamentous injury and for injuries of the posterolateral structures. For the posterior cruciate ligament acute operative repair is preferable, as a delay in treatment is associated with poor results. However, acute repair is not always successful.
Follow-up treatment: A hinged knee brace for 6–8 weeks followed by exercises with focus on restoring muscle strength.

Duration
Injury takes 6–8 weeks to heal.
Duration of disability is 3–12 weeks.

Prognosis
The posterior drawer test often remains positive after reconstruction. Results of secondary posterior cruciate ligament reconstruction are poor. When instability persists, problems in the patellofemoral area often occur. However, good function and well trained muscles can greatly compensate for the instability.

10.10   Meniscus injuries

Mechanism of injury
Rotational force impacts the flexed loaded knee, usually during sports or after a fall. Most meniscus injuries are of a degenerative nature.

Clinical presentation
With a peripheral tear, ie, acute pain in the knee, rapid swelling of the joint, and the knee cannot take a load in extension. Pain in the medial or lateral aspect. A displaced meniscus can lead to a locked knee, meaning the knee cannot be extended but it can be flexed.

Diagnostics
Physical examination: For a peripheral tear: hemarthrosis, pain over the lateral or medial joint line, pain on flexion, extension, and rotation. With nonperipheral longitudinal tears, acute hemarthrosis does not necessarily occur. A "bucket handle" injury can lead to a locked knee (Fig 10-15e).

X-ray examination: X-rays of the knee in two planes to exclude bone injuries.

Other examinations: When meniscus injury is strongly suspected perform an MRI or arthroscopy which can include a curative intervention. If problems persist, atrophy of the thigh musculature occurs. Arthrography may be useful if MRI is limited by metallic artifact from nearby implants.

Classification (Fig 10-15)
- Injury of the medial or the lateral meniscus
- Peripheral longitudinal tear
- Horizontal tear
- Bucket handle tear
- Degenerative tear

The accurate traumatic meniscus injury is a peripheral tear, often in combination with tendon or cruciate ligament injuries. Most longitudinal tears of the meniscus are the result of existing degenerative abnormalities.

Treatment
Conservative treatment: For partial tears of the outer margin of the meniscus, often occurring in combination with minimal ligamentous injury, and in degenerative tears causing few symptoms.

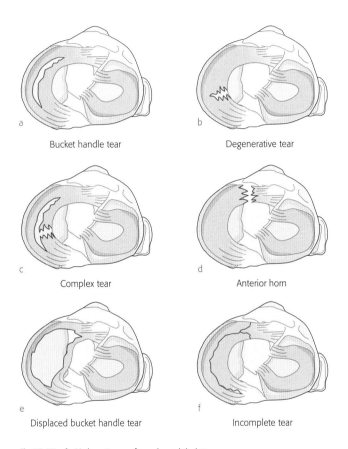

a   Bucket handle tear

b   Degenerative tear

c   Complex tear

d   Anterior horn

e   Displaced bucket handle tear

f   Incomplete tear

Fig 10-15a–f Various types of meniscus injuries.

Surgical treatment: An isolated meniscus injury seldom requires acute surgery, unless associated with restrictions in extension. A large peripheral tear, in the vascularized peripheral 1/3, can best be repaired within 14 days. Because this sort of tear is often associated with injuries to the collateral ligament and/or cruciate ligament, insertion of the meniscus to the ligament and/or tendon attachment itself, respectively, should be performed at the same time.

Follow-up treatment: After repairing the meniscus use a cast or brace for 6 weeks, restricting the extremes of flexion/extension. Muscle exercises supervised by a physiotherapist.

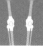

Duration
After suturing of the meniscus the injury takes 8 weeks to heal; after partial meniscectomy, 3–4 weeks.
Duration of disability is 6–8 weeks after suturing of the meniscus; after partial meniscectomy, 3–4 weeks.

Prognosis
Prognosis of isolated meniscus injury in patients with a normal leg axis is good with regard to the function of the leg. When related to other abnormalities, the prognosis depends more on other structures than on the meniscus itself. After total meniscectomy, the risk of arthrosis is high. Since the introduction of arthroscopy, total meniscectomy is rarely if ever indicated.

10.11   Knee dislocation

Mechanism of injury
Rotational trauma of the affected knee with a load to the leg. Violent direct or indirect force with a varus or valgus component. Generally caused by a motor vehicle injury, fall from height, or sporting injury.

Clinical presentation
The entire knee is painful; swelling. No obvious deformity if the dislocation is reduced "spontaneously." The leg cannot take a load, particularly in extension. Obvious displacement of the tibia in relation to the femur in dislocated position (Fig 10-16).

Diagnostics
Physical examination: There is often no hemarthrosis because blood seeps out of the torn soft tissues. Pain exists on all movements, mainly on valgus and varus stress and rotation. When the knee is dislocated, all movement is impossible. A thorough neurological and vascular examination is essential.

- Dislocation can resolve spontaneously.

- Neurovascular injury is common.

X-ray examination: X-rays of the knee in two planes.
Other examinations: Test the stability with the patient anesthetized; angiography or ankle-brachial pressure measurements (< 0.8 is significant for possible arterial injury). An MRI is useful to identify all injured structures.

Classification

Classification according to instability:

- Dislocation
- Anteromedial instability
- Anterolateral instability
- Posterolateral instability

Treatment

Conservative treatment: The dislocated knee must be reduced at once by traction, pressure is applied to the displaced tibia. Arterial injury must be ruled out.

Surgical treatment: When reduction fails and if there are problems with circulation. With anteromedial or anterolateral instability, surgical repair of the damaged structures is indicated. Attention must be paid to the posterolateral and posteromedial structures, the collateral ligaments, the capsule, and the menisci. With posterolateral instability, repair of the posterolateral structures and/or the posterior cruciate ligament can be considered.

Follow-up treatment: After conservative therapy use a cast or brace for 4–6 weeks. Next, careful mobilization with a CPM device. After surgical treatment use a brace with restricted flexion and extension for 6 weeks to 3 months, combined with physiotherapy, especially muscle-strengthening exercises.

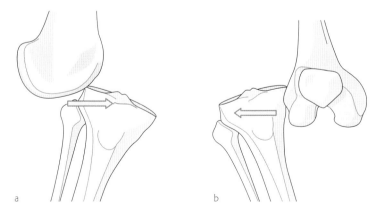

Fig 10-16a–b   Knee dislocation: a anterior dislocation; b lateral dislocation.

Duration

Injury takes 3–6 months to heal.

Duration of disability is 3–6 months, depending on the load to the leg. With a sedentary occupation, work can be started earlier.

Prognosis

Prognosis is reasonable if a good stability is achieved and the muscular strength is good.

10.12   Tibial eminence (spine) fractures

Mechanism of injury

Forced flexion or hyperextension of the knee. The cruciate ligaments remain intact, and a pull off of their insertion into the proximal tibia occurs usually in adolescents (Figs 10-17, 10-18).

■ This injury is usually equivalent to injuries of the anterior cruciate ligament.

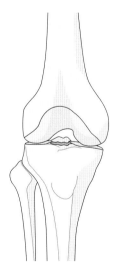

Fig 10-17   Fracture of the tibial eminentia without displacement.

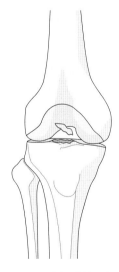

Fig 10-18   Fracture of the tibial eminentia with displacement.

Clinical presentation

Pain, swelling, and restriction on extension; weight bearing is not possible with the leg extended. The knee is held in flexion.

Diagnostics

Physical examination: Hemarthrosis, restriction and pain on extension, laxity in AP direction with good collateral stability.

X-ray examination: X-rays of the knee in two planes, combined with a tunnel view; CT scan or tomography may be used to determine the extent of the fracture.

Classification

- Nondisplaced fracture
- Fracture with marginal displacement that can be reduced by extending the leg
- Displaced (irreducible) fracture

Treatment

Conservative treatment: If good reduction can be obtained with the knee extended in a cast.

Surgical treatment: For persistent displacement use fixation by means of osteosynthesis, screw, or tension suture which may be performed by arthroscopy.

Follow-up treatment: 4–5 weeks in a cast followed by mobilizing exercises and temporary protection in a brace. Muscle-strengthening exercises.

Duration

Injury takes 6 weeks to heal.
Duration of disability is 8 weeks.

Prognosis

Prognosis is good.

10.13 Tibial plateau fractures

Mechanism of injury
Considerable direct force in valgus or varus position. An isolated impression of the plateau can occur without appreciable displacement. A serious fall can lead to a double impression with multiple fragments and a Y-fracture of the proximal tibia. Soft tissues can be seriously injured.

Clinical presentation
Pain in the knee, also the proximal part of the tibia with swelling of the joint; weight bearing is not possible. Abnormal axis.

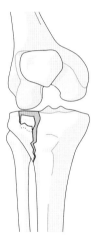

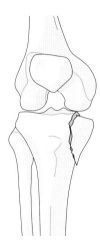

Fig 10-19   Fracture of the lateral part of the tibial plateau with depression.

Fig 10-20   Fracture of the medial part of the tibial plateau.

Diagnostics
Physical examination: Pain of the medial or lateral aspect of the knee joint at the level of the proximal tibia. Hemarthrosis is not always present because blood seeps into the surrounding tissues. All movements are painful. Varying degrees of instability depend on the size of displaced fragments.

X-ray examination: X-rays of the knee in two planes; oblique views, CT scan, or tomography is useful to determine the severity of the fracture and the position of fracture parts.

Classification

- Lateral plateau fracture (Fig 10-19)
- Medial plateau fracture (Fig 10-20)
- Y-fracture
- Depression fracture (Fig 10-19)
- Split fracture
- Combination fracture (Fig 10-21)

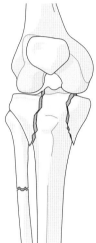

Fig 10-21   Fracture of the tibial plateau involving both the medial and lateral condyles of the tibia.

When choosing treatment, it is important to determine whether depression of one or both parts of the plateau is also associated with comminution and whether the periphery of the plateau blocks is reasonably intact. Sometimes the injury is associated with a fracture of the fibular head or neck.
Müller AO Classification: 41-B(1–3) or 41-C(1–3).

- Watch out for soft-tissue injuries.

Treatment
Conservative treatment: If there is no damage to the ligamentous structures, if the tibia is not displaced, and if the knee is stable with varus/valgus testing in extension use functional treatment in a hinged knee brace or a cast for 6 weeks; avoid weight bearing by using crutches.

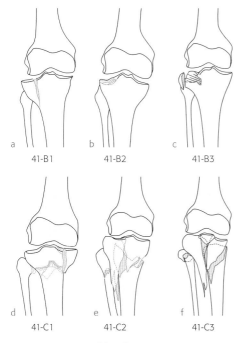

Fig 10-22a–f   Müller AO Classification of types B and C fractures of the proximal tibia.

- In patients older than 60 years an impression fracture 10 mm or less may be treated conservatively, provided the knee is stable in extension.

Surgical treatment: For serious depression of one or both of the plateau halves resulting in instability use reduction of the plateau with cancellous bone grafting or use a bone substitute to fill in the resulting bone defect under arthroscopic monitoring or by arthrotomy. With fractures of the peripheral osseous structures treatment consists of fixation with osteosynthesis material, usually screws with or without a supporting plate (Fig 10-23).

- Accompanying injury of the meniscus is frequent. Repair is usually possible.

Follow-up treatment: After surgery, functional treatment or CPM. If good mobility is achieved in combination with adequate muscular control and secure fixation, partial weight bearing is allowed using crutches after 6–8 weeks. Also exercise therapy with focus on restoring muscular strength.

Duration
Injury takes 6 weeks to 3 months to heal.
Duration of disability is 6 weeks to 6 months.

Prognosis
Prognosis depends on the degree to which the anatomical proportions can be restored (congruity, stability, and axial alignment). With persisting articular irregularities and/or instability, the risk of arthrosis is high. If the axial deviation is not restored to normal, there is a high risk of unicompartmental arthrosis.

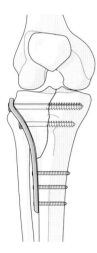

Fig 10-23   Monocondylar fracture of the tibial plateau treated with lag screws and plate as support.

10.14   Tibial tuberosity fractures

Mechanism of injury
Direct force from direct trauma to the anterior aspect of the knee or indirect force involving impact to the patellar tendon.

Clinical presentation
Swelling at the level of the tibial tuberosity which can be related to hemarthrosis. Weight bearing is painful and it is impossible to lift the extended leg.

■ This injury usually occurs in adolescents. It is an epiphyseal fracture, Salter-Harris type III (Fig 10-25).

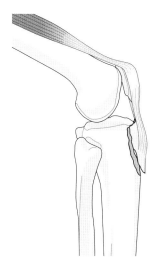

Fig 10-24 Avulsion of the tibial tuberosity.

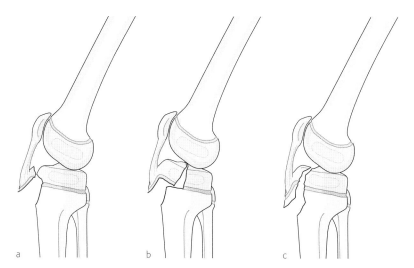

a   b   c

Fig 10-25a–c   Injuries of the epiphysis of the proximal tibia in children, Salter-Harris types I, III, and IV by traction of the patellar tendon. a Fracture through apophysis at insertion of patella tendon; b Salter-Harris type III; c Salter-Harris type IV.

Diagnostics
Physical examination: Local swelling and pain at the level of the tibial tuberosity, hemarthrosis, good AP, and collateral stability. It is not possible to lift the extended leg.
X-ray examination: X-rays of the knee in two planes.

■ Consider the possibility of Osgood-Schlatter disease.

Classification
■ Intraarticular fractures
■ Extraarticular fractures
Or the classification according to Ogden with three main types, each with two subtypes, depending on localization, displacement, or comminution.

Treatment
Conservative treatment: In adults if anatomical reduction of the tuberosity is possible use a cast for 6 weeks.
Surgical treatment: Fixation with a screw and/or a tension band.
Follow-up treatment: After short-lasting exercises, a cast or brace for 6 weeks with weight bearing in extension only.

Duration
Injury takes 6 weeks to heal.
Duration of disability is approximately 6 weeks.

Prognosis
Prognosis is good.

10.15 Fractures of epiphysis of the proximal tibia

Mechanism of injury
Indirect force with valgus or varus stress to an epiphysis that has not yet closed.

Clinical presentation
Pain in and around the knee with axial deviation; weight bearing is not possible.

Diagnostics
Physical examination: Swelling in and around the joint, lateral instability, hemarthrosis only with Salter-Harris types III and IV injuries.

■ With severe displacement check for neurovascular injuries.

X-ray examination: X-rays of the knee in two planes; the epiphysiolysis and displacement of the osseous structures are usually visible. Sometimes the epiphysiolysis can only be seen on x-ray in varus and valgus stress with the patient anesthetized.

Classification
According to Salter-Harris (see chapter 3 Principles of fracture treatment):
Type I: Fracture through zone of ossification
Type II: Fracture through zone of ossification with metaphyseal fragment
Type III: Epiphyseal fracture (Fig 10-26)
Type IV: Epiphyseal fracture extending to the metaphysis
Type V: Compression of the growth plate

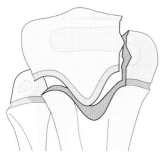

Fig 10-26   Injuries of the metaphysis of the proximal tibia, Salter-Harris type III.

Treatment
Conservative treatment: If anatomical reduction is achieved use a circular long-leg cast for 4–6 weeks.
Surgical treatment: If reduction is not successful or if there are doubts about the interposition of soft tissues; treatment consists of open reduction and osteosynthesis without damaging the growth zone.
Follow-up treatment: Short mobilization using a CPM device, followed by a cast for 6 weeks.

Duration
Injury takes 6 weeks to heal.

Prognosis
Prognosis is good when anatomical proportions are restored. If the growth zone is damaged, axial abnormalities can occur; thus requiring secondary correction.

10.16 Fibular head dislocation

Mechanism of injury
Indirect force caused by a fall from height, landing on the inverted foot in plantar flexion with the knee bent. Direct force to the external aspect of the lower leg at the level of the fibular head connected to a rupture of the proximal syndesmosis.

Clinical presentation
Acute pain of the external aspect of the lower leg at the level of the knee and the fibular head. Weight bearing is possible but movements are painful.

- Assess for paralysis of muscles supplied by the peroneal nerve, and check for sensory abnormalities in the lower leg and foot.

- Be alert for injuries to the ankle joint with diastasis of the ankle mortise (see chapter 11 Ankle and foot injuries).

Diagnostics
Physical examination: Local swelling, hematoma, and pain on loading and on attempts to move the fibular head. Inversion, eversion, and lifting the foot are painful at the level of the proximal fibula.
X-ray examination: X-rays of the knee in two planes, including the whole of the lower leg and ankle. The AP and lateral views show displacement and direction of the displacement, respectively.

Classification

Harrison classification according to the direction of the displacement:

- Anterolateral (Fig 10-27a–b)
- Dorsal (Fig 10-27c–d)
- Proximal (always related to ankle injury or in combination with a tibial fracture) (Fig 10-27e–f)

Treatment

Conservative treatment: In acute cases use closed reduction, immobilization with a cast for 5 weeks. If the fibular head proves to be stable after reduction use an elastic bandage.

Surgical treatment: In delayed or unrecognized cases when a clear dislocation of the fibular head occurs during certain movements and/or can be manipulated—fixation of the fibula to the tibia with a plasty, using part of the biceps tendon of the femur in combination with a screw. An alternative is arthrodesis of the proximal tibiofibular joint.

Follow-up treatment: A cast for 5 weeks.

Duration

Injury takes 5–6 weeks to heal.
Duration of disability is 6 weeks.

Prognosis

Prognosis is good.

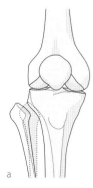
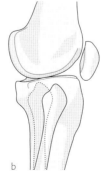

Fig 10-27a–f   Classification of dislocations of the fibular head according to Harrison.
a–b Anterolateral dislocation of fibular head.

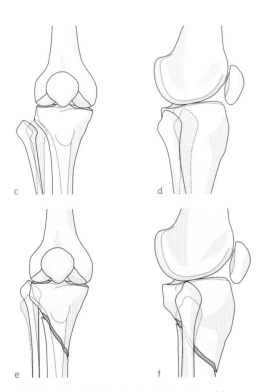

Fig 10-27a–f (cont) Classification of dislocations of the fibular head according to Harrison. c–d Dorsal dislocation of fibular head. e–f Dislocation in combination with proximal tibial shaft fracture.

10.17   Fibular shaft fractures

Mechanism of injury
Direct force to the lateral aspect of the lower leg.

Clinical presentation
Pain at the external aspect of the lower leg with slight swelling.

- Check for accompanying injury to the ankle (see chapter 11 Ankle and foot injuries).

Diagnostics
Physical examination: Pain on palpation of the fibula.

- Accompanying ankle injuries should be excluded.

X-ray examination: X-rays of the whole of the lower leg in two planes, so including the knee and ankle.

Classification
Distinction should be made between a fibular fracture by direct force without further damage and a fibular fracture linked to ankle injuries.

Treatment
No specific treatment in isolated fractures, return to normal activities as pain permits.

- Check for accompanying ankle injury.

Duration
Injury takes 4–6 weeks to heal.
Duration of disability is 2–6 weeks.

Prognosis
Prognosis is good.

10.18 Tibial and fibular shaft fractures (fractura cruris)

Mechanism of injury

Indirect or direct injury during sport, a motor vehicle injury, or a fall from height. Often consists of a rotational component.

Clinical presentation

Swelling of the lower leg at the fracture site and severe pain; weight bearing is not possible. Depending on the site of the fracture, movement of the knee or ankle is usually painful. Sometimes there is an obvious deformity.

Diagnostics

Physical examination: Bruising or abrasions of the covering skin with severe hematoma formation. All movements and load to the leg are painful. Obvious deformity.

X-ray examination: X-rays of the whole of the lower leg in two planes, including the knee and ankle.

- Check for neurovascular injuries.

- Compartment syndrome may occur.

Classification

Shaft fractures are classified according to localization, degree of displacement, single or multiple, and comminuted, open or closed. The condition of soft tissues and mainly the skin is significant.

Müller AO Classification: 42-A, 42-B, and 42-C with fibular fracture (Fig 10-28).

Treatment

Conservative treatment: In nondisplaced fractures or if simple reduction can produce a stable position use a cast or brace for 8–12 weeks. Shortening of 1 cm is acceptable (Fig 10-29).

- A good soft-tissue covering of the fracture is essential for rapid healing.

- Check for axial and rotational deviation.

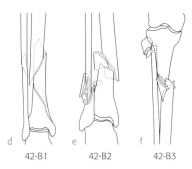

a 42-A1　b 42-A2　c 42-A3　d 42-B1　e 42-B2　f 42-B3

g 42-C1　h 42-C2　i 42-C3

Fig 10-28a–i　Müller AO Classification of fractures of the tibial and fibular shaft.

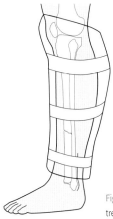

Fig 10-29　Fracture of the tibial shaft treated with a brace.

Surgical treatment: In unstable (displaced) fractures where the axis cannot be maintained, and in fractures connected to serious soft-tissue injuries. The choice of surgical method depends on the preferences and experience of the treating surgeon. A locked intramedullary nail is most often used (Fig 10-30). In isolated tibial shaft fractures nonoperative treatment is indicated in undisplaced fractures.

- Isolated tibial shaft fractures may slowly develop a varus deformity—close x-ray follow-up is indicated.

- Isolated tibial shaft fractures may be slow to unite.

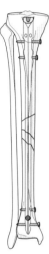

Fig 10-30   Fracture of the tibial shaft treated with a locked intramedullary nail.

Duration
Injury takes 6–16 weeks to heal.
Duration of disability is 12–24 weeks.

Prognosis
Prognosis is good and is mainly determined by accompanying injuries to soft tissues and/or any complications that may develop.

10.19 Achilles tendon rupture

Mechanism of injury
Indirect trauma from an acute powerful contraction of the calf muscles, usually during sport caused by pushing off or abrupt movement. There is nearly always a preexisting degeneration of the tendon.

Clinical presentation
A typical patient is between 30 and 45 years' old. Often an audible pop is heard, followed by pain, swelling over the Achilles tendon, and the inability to walk properly and stand on tiptoe. Patients feel as if they have been kicked from behind.

Diagnostics
Physical examination: Pain over the Achilles tendon with local swelling and a palpable dent in the tendon, 4–6 cm above the calcaneus (Fig 10-31). Inability to be on tiptoe and walk properly. Thompson sign (Simmonds test) is positive (Fig 10-32); squeezing calf muscles causes plantar flexion of the foot if the Achilles tendon is intact or partially torn but not if there is a complete rupture of the tendon.
X-ray examination: MRI or ultrasound can be useful to verify a partial tear.

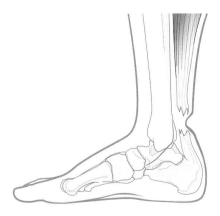

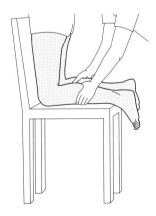

Fig 10-31   Dent as a result of a rupture of the Achilles tendon.

Fig 10-32   Thompson test.

Classification
None; partial ruptures are rare.

Treatment
Conservative treatment: Long-leg cast with the foot in an equinus position for 6 weeks. Next, the foot is gradually brought out of equinus and progressive partial weight-bearing exercises are started. Alternatively, a walking boot incorporating an adjustable heel may be used. With conservative treatment the risk of a rerupture is 5–15%.

Surgical treatment: Coaptation of the ruptured parts of the tendon, fixing them together or fixing the proximal part of the tendon to the calcaneus so that cast immobilization is not necessary. A 3-flap technique is often used. For missed or old cases, plasties are often possible. The most common complication is problems with wound healing. The risk of another rupture is less than 5% (Fig 10-33).

Follow-up treatment: Choice of cast immobilization or functional treatment (with or without tape bandage), depending on the surgical technique used.

Duration
Injury takes 6–8 weeks to heal.

Duration of disability is strongly dependent on the patient's occupation (in some professions it is possible to work in a plaster cast) and lasts 2–12 weeks.

Prognosis
Prognosis is good; some increase in the size of the Achilles tendon, calf muscle atrophy, and slight shortening of the leg is possible.

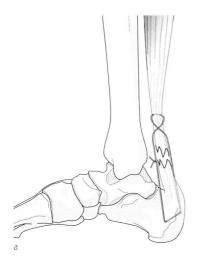

a

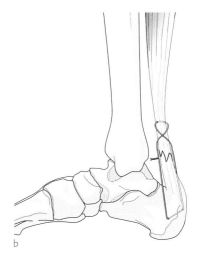

b

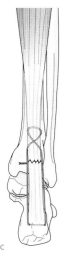

c

Fig 10-33a–c   Treatment of Achilles tendon rupture with fixation of the proximal part of the tendon to the calcaneus.

11   Ankle and foot injuries

11.1   Rupture of tibiofibular syndesmosis

Mechanism of injury
Indirect trauma caused by forced eversion/external rotation. This injury rarely occurs on its own.

Clinical presentation
Pain and swelling of the anterior aspect of the lower leg, just above the ankle joint. Weight bearing is possible but painful.

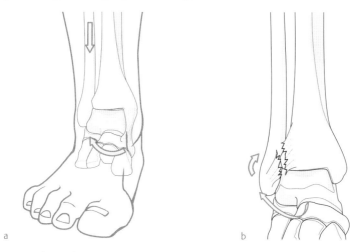

a   b

Fig 11-1a–b   Mechanism of injury of a rupture of the anterior syndesmosis.

Diagnostics
Physical examination: Local pain on palpation at the level of the anterior syndesmostic ligament. Occasionally local tenderness at the level of the medial malleolus.

X-ray examination: X-rays of the ankle and the lower leg in two planes to exclude an avulsion fracture (Tillaux fracture). Widening of the distal tibio-fibular joint with or without a fracture of the fibular shaft (Maisonneuve fractures) (Fig 11-1).

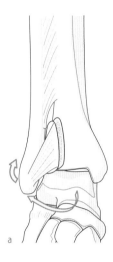

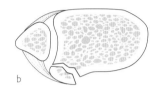

Fig 11-2a–b   Avulsion fracture of the anterior syndesmotic ligament at its tibial insertion (Tillaux-Chaput tubercle).

Classification
None.

Treatment
Conservative treatment: First reduce the swelling with ice packs and a pressure bandage. A splint is sometimes used to ease pain and prevent equinus. Tape bandage after 5–7 days and start weight bearing straight away with the patient wearing sports shoes.

Surgical treatment: For stable injuries reduce the dislocation and stabilize the joint with a positioning screw inserted between the fibula and tibia above the inferior tibiofibular joint.

Duration
Injury takes 4–6 weeks to heal.
Duration of disability is 6 weeks.

Prognosis
Prognosis is good if stability is restored.

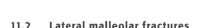

11.2 Lateral malleolar fractures

Mechanism of injury
Failure in tension with foot supinated and adduction force applied. A direct blow is a rare occurrence (Fig 11-3).

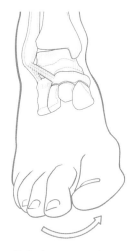

Fig 11-3   Mechanism of injury of an inversion injury of the ankle.

Clinical presentation
Pain on or behind the fibula, local swelling, and hemarthrosis. Weight bearing is possible but painful.

Diagnostics
Physical examination: Local pain on palpation of the distal fibula, diffuse swelling, characteristic fracture symptoms, deformity of the foot with severe displacement.
X-ray examination: X-rays in two planes with AP view in 20° internal rotation.

Classification
- Injury of the epiphyseal plate in a child.
- Avulsion fracture, corresponding to an injury of the lateral ligament.
- As part of a fracture dislocation of the ankle joint, Danis-Weber classification according to position of the fracture in relation to the syndesmosis. The stability of the syndesmosis is determined by the level of the injury. The syndesmosis is never disrupted in type A, often disrupted in type B, and

always disrupted in type C injuries. This distinction forms part of the Müller AO Classification (Fig 11-7).

- Failure of lateral malleolus foot in supination resulting in talar tilt and external rotation (Fig 11-4d–f).
- Failure of malleolus with foot in pronation while an external rotation force is applied (Fig 11-4g–j).

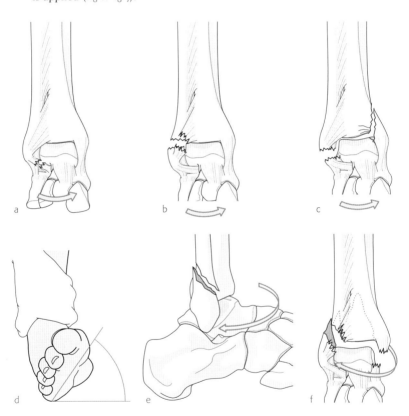

Fig 11-4a–j   a Rupture of anterior talofibular ligament. b Transverse fibular avulsion fracture. c Avulsion fracture of the fibula and vertical fracture of medial malleolus. d Mechanism of injury (supinated foot). e External rotation of talus causes spiral fracture of lateral malleolus. f Further talar rotation causes fractures of the posterior articular up of the tibia (Vollmann triangle) and medial failure, ie, rupture of deltoid ligament or fracture of medial malleolus.

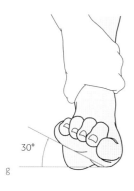

30°

g

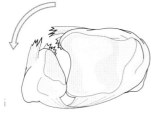

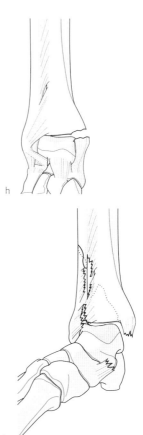

i

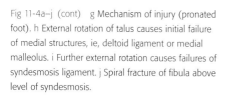

Fig 11-4a–j (cont) g Mechanism of injury (pronated foot). h External rotation of talus causes initial failure of medial structures, ie, deltoid ligament or medial malleolus. i Further external rotation causes failures of syndesmosis ligament. j Spiral fracture of fibula above level of syndesmosis.

j

A fracture of the fibula can be isolated, but it is usually part of a complex and therefore unstable ankle injury. Unstable injuries of the fibular shaft can be associated with:

- Rupture of the deltoid ligament (unimalleolar fractures)
- Fracture of the medial malleolus (bimalleolar fracture)
- Fracture of the medial malleolus and of the posterior malleolus (trimalleolar fractures)

Treatment

Conservative treatment: For Salter-Harris types I (Fig 11-5) and II injuries use short-leg walking cast for 6 weeks. For an isolated Weber type A injury use a short-leg walking cast for 4–6 weeks; functional treatment using a tape bandage is also possible. For an isolated (stable) Weber type B injury use a walking cast for 6 weeks after reduction.

Surgical treatment: For Weber type A injuries associated with a fracture dislocation of the ankle joint use screws or tension band. For Weber type B injuries (Fig 11-6) if the talus is laterally displaced in the ankle mortise use lag screws or osteosynthesis with plate and screws. For Weber type C injuries (Fig 11-8) use osteosynthesis with plate and screws and/or positioning screw (a screw inserted through the fibula and tibia to stabilize the inferior tibiofibular joint; then nonweight-bearing ambulation, with crutches or a walking cast for 6 weeks.

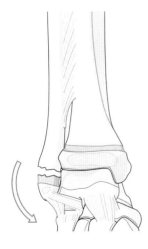

Fig 11-5   Epiphysiolysis of the lateral malleolus in a child, Salter-Harris type I.

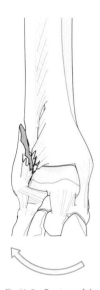

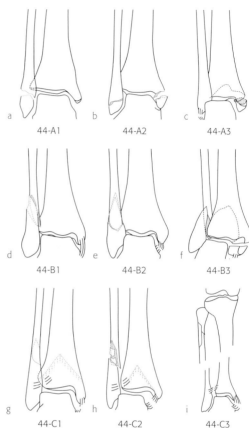

Fig 11-6 Fracture of the lateral malleolus, Weber type B as a result of supination and eversion.

44-A1 44-A2 44-A3

44-B1 44-B2 44-B3

44-C1 44-C2 44-C3

Fig 11-7a–i Müller AO Classification of ankle fractures; type 44-C3 is the so-called Maisonneuve fracture: high fracture of the fibula or fibular head dislocation with rupture of the interosseous membrane.

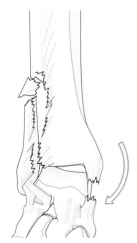

Fig 11-8 Fracture of the lateral malleolus, Weber type C injury with rupture of the deltoid ligament as a result of abduction and external rotation with the foot in pronation.

Duration

Injury takes 6–8 weeks to heal.
Duration of disability is 8–12 weeks.

Prognosis

Prognosis depends on the type of injury. Weber type C injuries have the worst prognosis. There is a risk of early arthrosis of the ankle joint if an anatomical position is not achieved. Reduction in joint space can be seen in 30–50% of cases in x-rays taken 2 years after injury.

11.3   Medial malleolar fractures

Mechanism of injury

Indirect trauma caused by forced inversion/eversion and/or rotational injury at the level of the ankle joint. Direct force to the inferior aspect of the ankle.

Clinical presentation

Swelling over the medial malleolus; pain felt on the medial aspect of the ankle.

Diagnostics

Physical examination: Hemarthrosis of the ankle joint. Pain on palpation and on loading.

X-ray examination: X-rays of the ankle in two planes; additional x-rays may be needed in different degrees of rotation.

- Accessory ossicle may be seen on x-ray.

- Exclude Maisonneuve fracture.

Classification

- Avulsion fracture
- Transverse fracture, usually related to a bimalleolar or trimalleolar fracture—traction injury to the medial complex
- Vertical fracture (compression injury to the medial complex)

Treatment

Conservative treatment: A small avulsion fracture is treated as a ligamentous injury. First reduce the swelling with ice packs and a pressure bandage. A splint is sometimes used to ease pain and prevent equinus. Tape bandage after 5–7 days and start full weight bearing immediately, with the patient wearing sports shoes. The treatment of nondisplaced fractures consists of a short-leg cast for 6 weeks after reduction.

Surgical treatment: In displaced fractures use fixation with a tension band or screws. Then functional treatment, partial weight bearing with crutches, or a short-leg cast for 6 weeks.

Duration
Injury takes 6 weeks to heal in all cases.
Duration of disability is 6–8 weeks.

Prognosis
Prognosis is good.

11.4   Posterior malleolar fractures

Mechanism of injury
A fall with the foot in maximal plantar flexion, or linked with a fracture dislocation of the ankle joint—a trimalleolar fracture (Figs 11-9, 11-10). Forced hyperextension as mechanism is extremely rare. Result is a small fracture fragment (Fig 11-11).

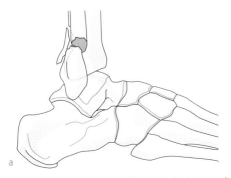

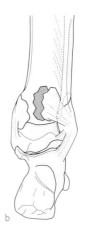

Fig 11-9a–b   a Spiral fracture of lateral malleolus caused by external rotation with foot in supination. b Talus rotates to hit past malleolus causing a fracture.

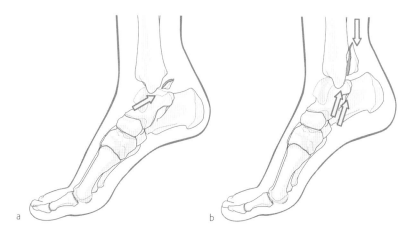

Fig 11-10a–b   Mechanism of injury of an isolated fracture of the posterior malleolus; the size of the fragment is determined by the direction of impact.

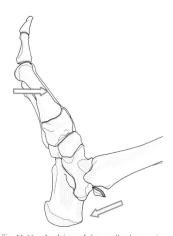

Fig 11-11   Avulsion of the malleolus tertius caused by hyperextension of the ankle.

Clinical presentation
Swelling of the ankle joint, pain on ambulation.

Diagnostics
Physical examination: Swelling, pain on palpation behind the medial malleolus. Pain on flexion/extension movements of the ankle joint.

X-ray examination: X-rays of the ankle in two planes. With a large fragment, dorsal subluxation of the talus occurs.

- An accessory ossicle is sometimes found at the posterior aspect of the tibia and talus.

- Always consider the possibility of a high fracture of the fibular shaft (Maisonneuve fracture).

Classification
None.

Treatment
Conservative treatment: For a small fragment and stable ankle apply functional therapy. Otherwise make use of closed reduction by dorsal extension of the ankle into an anatomical position. Next, a short-leg cast for 6 weeks with 3 weeks nonweight bearing, and then 3 weeks weight bearing.

Surgical treatment: With a step in the joint of more than 1 mm and/or a fragment larger than 1/3 of the joint area open reduction and screw fixation are essential. If the injury is related to a fibular fracture, anatomical reduction and fixation of the fibular fracture will usually reduce the posterior malleolar fracture by ligamentotaxis.

Follow-up treatment: Functional treatment, partial weight bearing using crutches or a short-leg cast for 6 weeks.

Duration
Injury takes 6 weeks to heal.
Duration of disability is 6–8 weeks.

Prognosis
There is a risk of posttraumatic arthrosis of the ankle if an anatomical position is not achieved.

11.5   Pilon fractures of the tibia

Mechanism of injury
Indirect trauma caused by a fall from height. Direct force from a motor vehicle injury.

Clinical presentation
Deformity, usually severe swelling around the ankle. Risk of a compromised blood supply to the skin or superficial soft-tissue injuries. Weight bearing is not possible.

Diagnostics
Physical examination: All signs of fracture.
X-ray examination: X-rays of the ankle in two planes. Sometimes three to four views are indicated in different degrees of rotation. A CT scan is very useful.

- Injury of the talus may occur.

- Can be associated with severe soft-tissue injury.

Classification
Classified in two types (Fig 11-12):
- With slight displacement
- Comminuted and displaced

Treatment
Surgical treatment: Open reduction and fixation of the fibula, reconstruction of the joint with cancellous bone grafting, and medial (and generally also lateral) support of the metaphyseal fracture. External fixation—crossing this ankle joint may be indicated if soft tissues are compromised. Because soft-tissue damage is severe in most of these injuries, definitive surgery is often best delayed to allow recovery of soft tissues. Use of a temporary spanning external fixator is helpful in such cases.

Duration
Injury takes 2–3 months to heal.
Duration of disability is 3–6 months.

Prognosis

Prognosis is poor for intraarticular comminuted fractures because of cartilaginous injury—early arthrosis of the upper tarsal joint often occurs. Consider arthrodesis if symptoms persist.

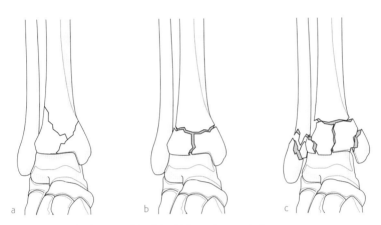

Fig 11-12a–c Pilon fractures of the tibia with increasing complexity.

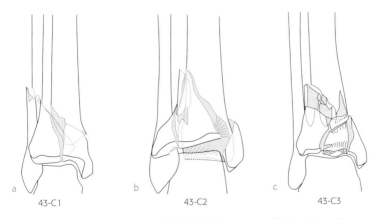

43-C1   43-C2   43-C3

Fig 11-13a–c Müller AO Classification of distal tibial fractures, type C (pilon fractures).

11.6   Injuries of the metaphysis of the distal tibia in children

Mechanism of injury
Bike injury in children, indirect trauma caused by rotational or loading forces during exercise, in traffic, or a fall.

Clinical presentation
Pain with weight bearing; sometimes a visible deformity is seen. This injury usually occurs in children aged 8–15 years.

Diagnostics
Physical examination: Swelling around the ankle, pain on palpation, and on loading.
X-ray examination: X-rays of the ankle in two planes, or CT scan.

Classification
Classification according to Salter-Harris:
Type I   Fracture through zone of ossification
Type II   Fracture through zone of ossification with metaphyseal fragment
           (Fig 11-14a)
Type III   Epiphyseal fracture (Fig 11-14b)
Type IV   Epiphyseal fracture extending to the metaphysis (Fig 11-14c)
Type V   Compression of the growth plate (Fig 11-14d)

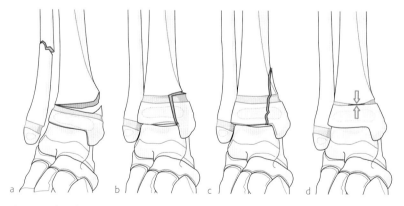

Fig 11-14a–d   Salter-Harris classification of metaphysis injuries of the distal tibia in children.
a Salter-Harris type II fracture. b Salter-Harris type III fracture. c Salter-Harris type IV fracture.
d Salter-Harris type V fracture.

Triplane fractures typically occur in the ankle (Fig 11-15); the two fractures ends on both sides of the metaphysis are perpendicular to each other (in adolescents at the end of the growth period before complete closure of the metaphysis).

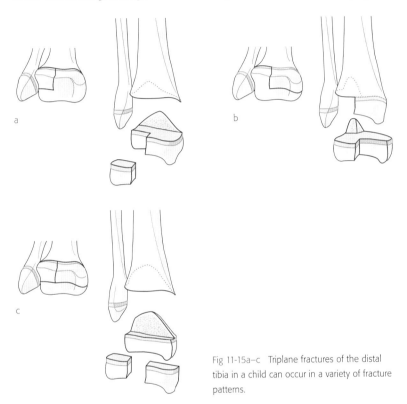

a

b

c

Fig 11-15a–c Triplane fractures of the distal tibia in a child can occur in a variety of fracture patterns.

Treatment

Conservative treatment: For Salter-Harris types I and II injuries—reduction if necessary, splint for 1 week, and then a short-leg cast for 5 weeks.

Surgical treatment: If closed reduction of Salter-Harris types I and II injuries is not successful, interposition of the periosteum has probably occurred. Treatment consists of open reduction and a cast or fixation with K-wires, a screw positioned parallel to the growth plate. For Salter-Harris type III injuries and in case of displacement of >2 mm use open reduction and screw fixation.

For Salter-Harris type IV injuries and triplane fractures—open reduction and fixation with screws parallel to the growth plate (Fig 11-16).

Follow-up treatment: A short-leg cast for 6 weeks, ie, 3 weeks nonweight bearing using crutches and 3 weeks weight bearing.

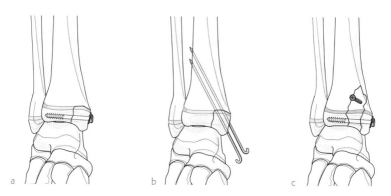

Fig 11-16a–c   Examples of internal fixation after anatomical reduction of epiphyseal fractures of the distal tibia in children.

Duration
Injury takes 6 weeks to heal.

Prognosis
Prognosis is good. If reduction of Salter-Harris types II and IV injuries is inadequate, there is a risk of early closure of the metaphysis resulting in growth arrest and axis abnormalities.

11.7   Peroneal tendon dislocation

Mechanism of injury
Indirect trauma from forced contraction of the peroneal muscles in an attempt to prevent acute inversion.

Clinical presentation
Acute pain and swelling over the distal end of the fibula. With recurrent dislocation, an audible, visible, and palpable tendon dislocation often occurs subcutaneously on active eversion.

Diagnostics

Physical examination: Swelling over the distal end of the fibula. Tenderness on palpation. The tendon can be palpated subcutaneously. Recurrent dislocation: on active eversion, the tendon displaces under the palpating finger.

- A diagnosis is rarely made in the acute phase.

X-ray examination: None.

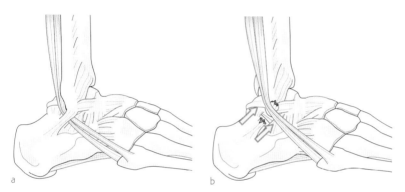

Fig 11-17a–b   Dislocation of peroneal tendons.

Classification

None.

Treatment

Surgical treatment: For new injuries use suturing of the peroneal tendon. For old injuries use rotation plasty according to Kelly (Fig 11-18) or reconstruction of soft tissues.
Follow-up treatment: A short-leg cast for 6 weeks.

Duration

Injury takes 6 weeks to heal.
Duration of disability is 6–8 weeks.

Prognosis

Prognosis is good.

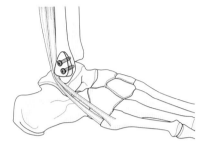

Fig 11-18   Peroneal tendon luxation treated with a Kelly plasty.

11.8   Rupture of the lateral collateral ligament of the ankle

Mechanism of injury

Indirect trauma from acute forced inversion of the ankle and foot (Fig 11-19).

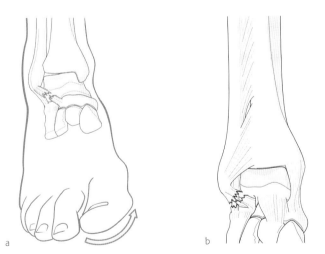

a   b

Fig 11-19a–b   Rupture of the lateral collateral ligaments of the ankle. a Anterior band only.
b Complete rupture.

Clinical presentation

Acute pain at the level of and distal to the lateral malleolus; local swelling. The patient is usually able to walk.

- 20% of patients complain of medial pain as a result of a local compression injury.

Diagnostics

Physical examination: Local hematoma, abnormal range of movement when the ankle is subjected to an inversion force. Talar tilt and anterior drawer test are difficult to achieve in the acute phase because of pain and active muscle resistance. Examination can be repeated after 5–7 days; ecchymosis occurs after 3–5 days.

- When there is pain on or behind the lateral malleolus, a fracture may have occurred. With pain distal to the fibula, consider a fracture of the base first.

X-ray examination (selective): X-rays of the ankle in two planes, only to exclude a fracture; take the AP view with 20° external rotation to enable good assessment of the talar dome.

- Osteochondral fracture of the talus may occur with lateral collateral ligament injuries (Fig 11-20).

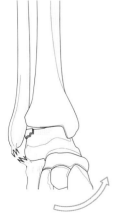

Fig 11-20   Mechanism of injury of an osteochondral fracture of the lateral talar margin.

■ Be aware that acute forced inversion may cause other injuries (Fig 11-21) which should be excluded by clinical examination.

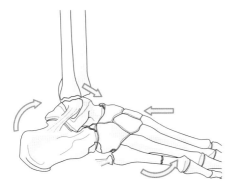

Fig 11-21 Various injuries that can occur with an acute forced inversion of the ankle and foot (supination line).

Classification
None. Although the lateral ankle ligament complex can be divided into three parts, this is not of any clinical significance because no relation has been shown between the extent of the ligamentous injury and the prognosis. Usually, only the anterior talofibular ligament is ruptured.

Treatment
Conservative treatment: First reduce swelling with ice packs and a pressure bandage. A splint is sometimes used to ease pain and prevent equinus. Tape bandage after 5–7 days and start full weight bearing straight away, with the patient wearing sports shoes for 3–6 weeks.
Surgical treatment: None.

Duration
Injury takes 3–6 weeks to heal.
Duration of disability is a few weeks for heavy manual work on uneven ground. It is possible for the patient to work while wearing a tape bandage. Sports can be restarted after 5–6 weeks.

Prognosis
The injury heals in 75% of patients without rest. The other 25% undergo mild instability problems. There is rarely an indication for secondary tendon plasty.

11.9 Rupture of the medial collateral ligament of the ankle

Mechanism of injury
Indirect trauma from acute forced eversion movement.

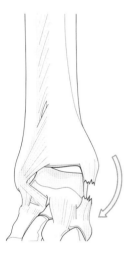

Fig 11-22 Rupture of the medial collateral ligament caused by acute forced eversion.

Clinical presentation
Local pain and swelling under the medial malleolus. The patient is able to walk. This injury is extremely rare.

Diagnostics
Physical examination: Local pain on palpation and swelling of the medial malleolus.
X-ray examination: X-rays of the ankle in two planes to exclude a fracture.

- Maisonneuve injury may occur with a high-fibular shaft fracture.

Classification
None. A distinction should be made between an isolated ligamentous injury (very rare) and a rupture in combination with a fibular fracture (Weber type B or C).

Treatment
Conservative treatment: Ice packs and a pressure bandage to reduce swelling. A splint is sometimes used to ease pain and prevent equinus. Tape bandage after 5–7 days and start full weight-bearing ambulation straight away, with the patient wearing sports shoes for 3 weeks.
Surgical treatment: None.

Duration
Injury takes 4–6 weeks to heal.
Duration of disability is a few weeks for heavy manual work on uneven ground. It is possible to work while wearing a tape bandage. Sports can be restarted after 5–6 weeks.

Prognosis
Prognosis is good.

11.10   Peripheral talar fractures

Mechanism of injury
Indirect trauma caused by inversion injury in combination with a rupture of the ankle ligament. Torsion force to the ankle joint.

Clinical presentation
Pain in the ankle on weight bearing. Immediate swelling of the ankle joint. Peripheral talus fractures are rare, and often presents as chronic ankle pain following a minor injury thought to be a "sprained ankle."

Diagnostics
Physical examination: Swelling, pain over the malleolus, either anterolaterally or posteromedially, depending on the site of the fracture. Pain with passive movement of the ankle.
X-ray examination: X-rays of the ankle in two planes, AP view in 20° external rotation.

■ Fractures of the posterior aspect of the talus can only be seen on an AP view of the ankle if the foot is in maximal plantar flexion. If in doubt, perform a CT scan or magnetic resonance imaging (MRI).

Classification

- Osteochondral fractures of the talar dome
- Fracture of the lateral process of the talus
- Fracture of the posterior process of the talus
- Fracture of the talar head

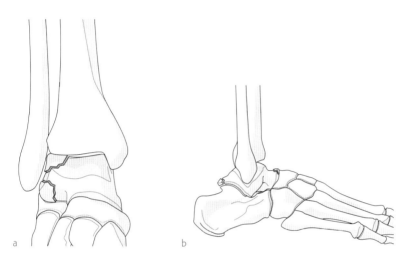

Fig 11-23a–b   Peripheral fractures of the talus.

Treatment

Conservative treatment: For small nondisplaced (osteochondral) fragments use a short-leg cast for 4 weeks, nonweight-bearing ambulation with crutches.

Surgical treatment: For a large-displaced fragment use arthrotomy, reduction, and (screw) fixation of the fragment. For a small displaced (osteochondral) fragment remove the fragment, by arthroscopy if necessary, and perform a microfracture technique (Fig 11-24).

Follow-up treatment: For a large fragment use functional treatment or a short-leg cast for 6 weeks, nonweight bearing with crutches. For a small-displaced fragment use functional treatment, start weight bearing as soon as possible.

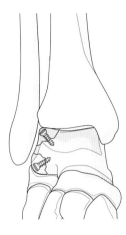

Fig 11-24   Peripheral fracture of the talus treated with a lag screw.

Duration
Injury takes 6 weeks to heal.
Duration of disability is 6–8 weeks.

Prognosis
Prognosis is good, unless a large (osteochondral) fragment needs to be removed or becomes fixed in a nonanatomical position; in such cases, there is a risk of early arthrosis.

11.11   Central talar fractures

Mechanism of injury
Indirect force, eg, fall from height. Direct force from a motor vehicle injury.

Clinical presentation
Weight bearing is not possible; swelling around the ankle joint.

Diagnostics
Physical examination: Hemarthrosis, pain on palpation around the ankle joint, and pain on passive movements of the ankle.
X-ray examination: X-rays of the ankle in two planes. If in doubt, perform a CT scan or MRI.

Classification
- Talar neck fracture with or without displacement
- Fracture of the talar body without displacement, with displacement, and comminuted

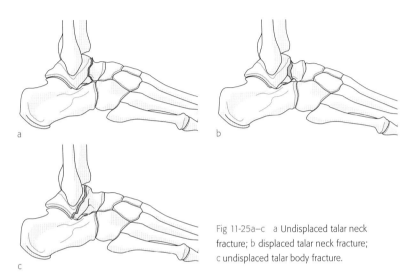

Fig 11-25a–c a Undisplaced talar neck fracture; b displaced talar neck fracture; c undisplaced talar body fracture.

Treatment
Conservative treatment: In nondisplaced fractures use short-leg cast with the ankle at 90° for 8 weeks, nonweight bearing.

Surgical treatment: Indicated with displacement, use open reduction and screw fixation (Figs 11-26, 11-27).

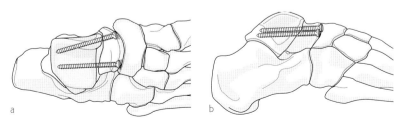

Fig 11-26a–b   Fracture of the talar neck with lag screws inserted dorsally.

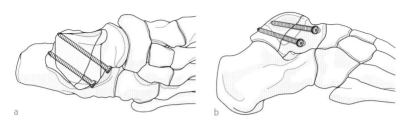

Fig 11-27a–b   Fracture of the talar body treated with lag screws.

■ Watch out for the congruity of the subtalar joint. With severe comminution: primary arthrodesis of the upper tarsal joint, maintaining the length may be indicated.

■ When operating, the delicate blood supply to the talus must be preserved.

Duration
Injury takes 8 weeks to 3 months to heal.
Duration of disability is 3–6 months.

Prognosis
The blood supply of the body of the talus comes from distal to proximal. Completely displaced fractures of the talar neck therefore may interrupt the blood supply to the body of the talus. Prognosis is uncertain owing to the risk of avascular necrosis of the talar body and the risk of arthrosis of the ankle or subtalar joints.

11.12   Dislocation and dislocation fractures of the talus

Mechanism of injury
Indirect trauma, eg, fall from height. Direct force from a motor vehicle injury. Forced plantar flexion.

Clinical presentation
Deformity of the ankle contour, often open soft-tissue injury on the medial aspect of the ankle, risk of compromised blood supply to the foot, and weight bearing is not possible.

Diagnostics

Physical examination: Severe swelling around the ankle joint, often with an abnormal contour and soft-tissue injury.

- Risk of skin damage and compartment syndrome of the foot if the injury is not treated promptly.

X-ray examination: X-rays of the ankle in two planes. As x-rays are sometimes difficult to interpret, repeat after reduction.

Classification

A distinction is made between a true dislocation of the talus and a fracture dislocation.

Dislocation:
- In the ankle joint (Fig 11-28)
- In the subtalar joint (Fig 11-29)
- Full talus dislocation (peritalar dislocation) (Fig 11-30)

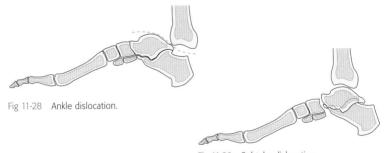

Fig 11-28   Ankle dislocation.

Fig 11-29   Subtalar dislocation.

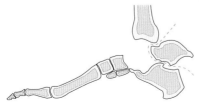

Fig 11-30   Peritalar dislocation.

- Subtalar (Fig 11-31)
- Midtarsal (Fig 11-32)
- "Aviators astragalus" (Fig 11-33)

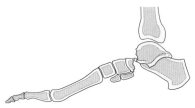

Fig 11-31   Subtalar dislocation fracture.

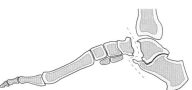

Fig 11-32   Midtarsal dislocation fracture.

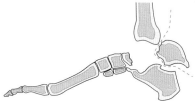

Fig 11-33   Aviators astragalus.

Treatment
Conservative treatment: For a dislocation use closed reduction and short-leg cast for 3–4 weeks and/or tape bandage. If closed reduction is not successful, open reduction using a medial malleolar osteotomy is indicated.
Surgical treatment: Indicated for a fracture dislocation—open reduction and screw fixation using anatomical reduction and lag screw fixation.

- Interposition of the tendon of the tibialis posterior tendon is possible, if reduction is not successful.

- Often circulation of the talar body only runs through the deltoid ligament.

Follow-up treatment: Nonweight bearing, with a short-leg cast or crutches for at least 6 weeks.

Duration
Injury takes 6 weeks to 3 months to heal.
Duration of disability is 3–6 months.

Prognosis
Prognosis is poor because of the risk of avascular necrosis of the talar body, and the risk of posttraumatic arthrosis of the ankle and subtalar joints.

11.13   Calcaneal fractures

Mechanism of injury
Direct force, eg, fall from height (Fig 11-34).

Clinical presentation
Pain, severe local swelling, and heel widening and shortening. The heel is in valgus and the longitudinal arch of the foot is flattened out.

Diagnostics
Physical examination: Pain on palpation of the heel bone. Severe swelling of soft tissues.
X-ray examination: X-rays in two planes (laterally and axially). Only perform a CT scan if surgery is being considered; tuberosity of the calcaneus is in inversion and shortened. There is comminution and widening of the lateral aspect; the sustentaculum tali is not displaced.

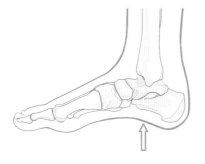

Fig 11-34   Mechanism of injury of a calcaneal fracture.

Classification

According to location:

- Peripheral avulsion (Fig 11-35a–b)
- Duck beak fracture (Fig 11-35c)
- Joint depression (Fig 11-35d)

According to complexity:

- Number of fragments
- Number of affected joints
- Degree of comminution

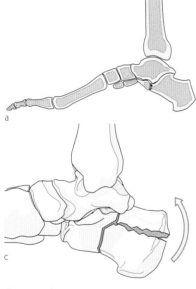

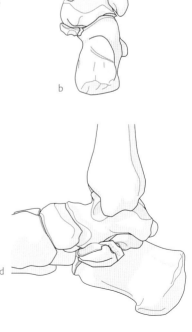

Fig 11-35a–d

a–b Peripheral avulsion fractures of the
   calcaneus: a anterior process;
   b sustentaculum tali.
c–d Central fractures of the calcaneus:
   c duck beak type; d joint area depression.

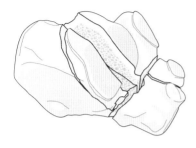

Fig 11-36   Comminuted intraarticular calcaneal fracture with depression of joint surface, incongruity, and widening.

Treatment

Conservative treatment: For nondisplaced body or avulsion fractures use short-leg cast for 4–6 weeks or functional treatment with tape bandage. For severe comminution in older patients or when there is vascular insufficiency (smokers or diabetics) use functional treatment. Nonweight bearing, with crutches for 6 weeks.

Surgical treatment: For duck beak fractures use tension band or screw fixation. A fracture with joint area depression is treated surgically in young, active patients to restore the contour of the foot and reconstruct the joint as well as possible (Fig 11-36). Treatment consists of reduction and fixation (plate, screws, K-wires).

Follow-up treatment: Nonweight bearing using crutches for 6–10 weeks. Then special shoes are sometimes necessary.

Duration

Injury takes 6–12 weeks to heal.
Duration of disability is 6–9 months.

Prognosis

Prognosis for displaced intraarticular fractures is poor. If special shoes are not effective, arthrodesis is indicated.

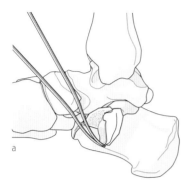

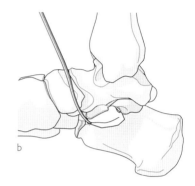

Fig 11-37a–b   Reduction of a tilted fragment carrying the joint related to a comminuted calcaneal fracture.

11.14   Cuboid bone fractures

Mechanism of injury
Direct force from a heavy object. Indirect trauma from acute forced abduction or inversion.

Clinical presentation
Pain and swelling of the lateral aspect of the tarsus. Pain on weight bearing.

Diagnostics
Physical examination: Swelling and local tenderness.
X-ray examination: X-rays in two planes, ie, an AP view of the tarsus and an oblique view. Comparative x-ray of the other foot is often necessary (Fig 11-38).

Classification
None.

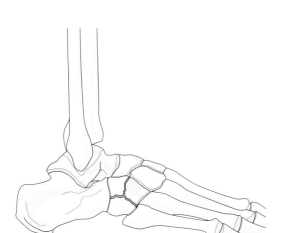

Fig 11-38 Cuboid fracture with three
fragments.

Treatment

Conservative treatment: For avulsion fractures linked to an injury to the supination line use functional treatment. First reduce swelling with ice packs and a pressure bandage. A splint is sometimes needed to ease pain and prevent equinus. Tape bandage after 5–7 days and start weight bearing straight away, with the patient wearing sports shoes for 3 weeks. For a minimally or nondisplaced fracture use short-leg cast for 4–6 weeks.

Surgical treatment: For displaced fractures with displacement of the fracture parts use open reduction and fixation with a screw or K-wire.

Follow-up treatment: Short-leg cast for 4–6 weeks.

Duration

Injury takes 4–6 weeks to heal.
Duration of disability is 6–8 weeks.

Prognosis

Prognosis is good if a good reduction is obtained. If symptoms persist and special shoes are not effective, arthrodesis is indicated.

11.15 Navicular bone fractures

Mechanism of injury
Indirect trauma caused by forced inversion/eversion of the foot. Forced plantar flexion of the foot.

Clinical presentation
Swelling of the tarsus, pain to the foot on weight bearing.

Diagnostics
Physical examination: Swelling and local tenderness.
X-ray examination: X-rays of the foot in two planes, ie, AP view and oblique view. Comparative x-rays of the other foot if necessary.

■ This fracture is often missed on x-ray. If in doubt, take more x-rays or perform a CT scan.

Classification
None.

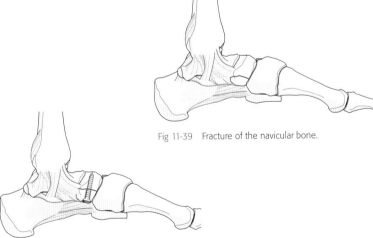

Fig 11-39   Fracture of the navicular bone.

Fig 11-40   Fracture of the navicular bone treated with a lag screw.

Treatment

Conservative treatment: In nondisplaced fractures: short-leg cast for 4–6 weeks (Fig 11-39).

Surgical treatment: For displaced fractures use open reduction and screw osteosynthesis, followed by nonweight-bearing ambulation with crutches or short-leg cast for 4 weeks (Fig 11-40).

Duration

Injury takes 4–6 weeks to heal.
Duration of disability is 6–8 weeks.

Prognosis

Prognosis is good. If symptoms persist and special shoes are not effective, arthrodesis of the surrounding joint(s) is indicated.

11.16 Fractures of metatarsals I–IV

Mechanism of injury

Direct force from a heavy object. Considerable axial load to the forefoot. Overloading (stress fracture).

Clinical presentation

The forefoot is diffusely swollen, weight bearing is painful.

Diagnostics

Physical examination: Pain of the forefoot at the level of the fracture on stressing the fracture site.

X-ray examination: X-rays of the foot in two planes with AP and oblique view. A fatigue fracture (March fracture) often cannot be seen on the first x-ray. A second set of films taken 2–3 weeks after onset of pain usually show profuse callus formation.

If there are clinical reasons for suspecting a fatigue fracture then bone scintigraphy or MRI can be performed if the x-ray shows no abnormalities (Fig 11-41).

■ Unexplained pain of the forefoot after exercise can point to a stress fracture.

Classification
None.

Treatment
Conservative treatment: For isolated fractures of metatarsals II, III, or IV use stiff-soled shoes. With severe pain or in case of a combination of fractures: short-leg cast for 4 weeks. For displaced fractures: closed reduction and cast.

Surgical treatment: For displaced fractures of metatarsal I because of the rolling function of the foot, use open reduction and fixation with screws or K-wires. For multiple-displaced fractures: open reduction and fixation with K-wires.

Follow-up treatment: Short-leg cast for 3 weeks, then remove K-wires.

Duration
Injury takes 4–6 weeks to heal.
Duration of disability is 6 weeks.

Prognosis
Prognosis is good; stiffness of the forefoot can persist if K-wires are inserted through the MTP joint.

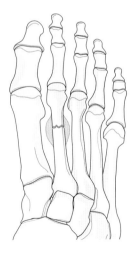

Fig 11-41 Fatigue fracture of the metatarsal bone II. After a few weeks, the fracture line and callus become visible.

11.17   Fractures of metatarsal V

Mechanism of injury

Acute forced adduction of the forefoot. This is an inversion injury.

Clinical presentation

Pain on the lateral side of the foot. Rolling the foot is painful. Initially, there is little swelling.

Diagnostics

Physical examination: Local tenderness at the base of metatarsal V. A hematoma only becomes visible after a few days.

X-ray examination: X-rays in two planes: AP and oblique views (Fig 11-42).

■ An avulsion fracture at the base of metatarsal V is often mistaken for a tear of the lateral collateral ligament ankle. A single x-ray will not show the injury.

■ In children, the epiphyseal plate should not be mistaken for an avulsion fracture.

Classification

- ■ Epiphysiolysis in adolescents
- ■ Avulsion fracture
- ■ Intraarticular fracture
- ■ Proximal fracture of the shaft (Jones fracture)

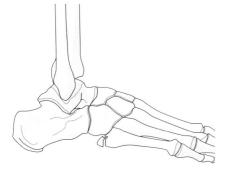

Fig 11-42   Avulsion fracture of the base of the fifth metatarsal can occur with acute forced inversion of the ankle and foot.

Treatment

Conservative treatment: For epiphysiolysis or an avulsion fracture apply functional treatment (tape bandage) for 4 weeks. For an isolated intraarticular fracture: walking cast or functional treatment for 4 weeks. For a proximal shaft fracture (Jones fracture): short-leg walking cast for 4–6 weeks.

Surgical treatment: Rarely indicated actively. The Jones fracture has a significant incidence of delay and nonunion. Persistent pain and absence of any signs of healing 6 weeks from injury are an indication for surgery using a lag screw.

Follow-up treatment: Nonweight-bearing ambulation with crutches or short-leg cast for 4 weeks.

Duration

Injury takes 4–6 weeks to heal.
Duration of disability is 4–6 weeks.

Prognosis

Prognosis is good for avulsion injuries.

■ Jones fractures are inclined to be related with pseudarthrosis formation (Fig 11-43).

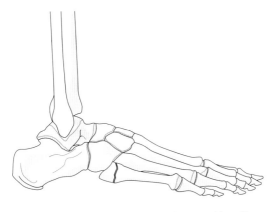

Fig 11-43 Proximal fracture of the shaft of metatarsal bone V (Jones fracture).

11.18 Midtarsal joint dislocation (Chopart joint)

Mechanism of injury
Direct trauma to the midfoot, forced plantar flexion. Forced inversion of the forefoot (in adduction or abduction); forced eversion of the midfoot.

Clinical presentation
Abnormal position of the forefoot with medial displacement, swelling of the dorsum of the midfoot, and pain on palpation.

Diagnostics
Physical examination: Swelling and pain of the midfoot.
X-ray examination: X-rays of the foot in two planes, AP and lateral views. If necessary, also oblique view.

Classification
According to the direction of the dislocation:
■ Medial
■ Lateral
■ Plantar

This dislocation is often linked to a fracture of the cuboid bone and/or the navicular bone.

Treatment
Conservative treatment: Is not indicated because of instability.
Surgical treatment: Closed reduction and percutaneous fixation using K-wires. When associated with a fracture of the cuboid bone and/or the navicular bone use open reduction and fixation of the fracture so that the dislocation reduces (spontaneously) and becomes stable.
Follow-up treatment: 4–6 weeks nonweight-bearing ambulation using crutches or a short-leg cast for 4 weeks. Then remove K-wires.

Duration
Injury takes 6 weeks to heal.
Duration of disability is 8–12 weeks.

Prognosis
There is a risk of midtarsal instability. If symptoms persist and special shoes are not effective, arthrodesis is indicated.

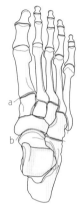

Fig 11-44   Foot skeleton
showing; a Chopart;
b Lisfranc joints.

11.19   Tarsometatarsal dislocation (Lisfranc joint)

Mechanism of injury
A fall on the foot in plantar flexion, forced hyperflexion/pronation of the forefoot. Direct force from a motor vehicle injury or locally from direct impact of a heavy object.

Clinical presentation
The foot is usually not able to support weight bearing; there is diffuse swelling of the forefoot. Often, a deformity of the forefoot in abduction is seen but swelling can disguise this.

- Check for soft-tissue injuries and compartment syndrome of the foot.

Diagnostics
Physical examination: Pain on palpation over the base of the metatarsals. Soft-tissue injury with severe swelling.

- Problems with blood supply to the forefoot can occur.

X-ray examination: X-rays of the midfoot in two planes. On AP view, the space between metatarsals I and II is widened. A CT scan provides additional information. True dislocations are rare; avulsions/fractures are nearly always at the base of the metatarsals.

■ This injury is not always correctly diagnosed from an x-ray; hence, it is not treated adequately.

Classification
■ Homolateral (Fig 11-45)
■ Isolated
■ Divergent (Fig 11-46)

Treatment
Conservative treatment: None. Closed reduction is inadequate because of instability from extensive injuries to the ligaments.
Surgical treatment: Closed reduction, percutaneous transarticular fixation with K-wires. Open reduction and transarticular screw fixation.
Follow-up treatment: Nonweight-bearing ambulation with short-leg cast for 4–6 weeks; then remove K-wires.

Duration
Injury takes 6 weeks to 3 months to heal.
Duration of disability is 3 months.

Prognosis
Prognosis is poor. There is a risk of stiffness owing to spontaneous arthrodesis. With inadequate reduction abduction of the forefoot occurs, causing pain on rolling the foot: special shoes or correction of arthrodesis is then required. A missed injury has a poor prognosis.

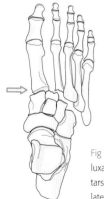

Fig 11-45 Example of luxation fracture of the tarsometatarsal (homolateral).

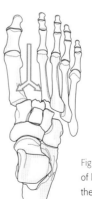

Fig 11-46 Example of luxation fracture of the tarsometatarsal (divergent).

11.20 Toes dislocation

Mechanism of injury
Direct force to the forefoot.

Clinical presentation
Pain, swelling. Deformity of the affected toe.

Diagnostics
Physical examination: Swelling, local tenderness. Few obvious abnormalities are usually seen.
X-ray examination: X-rays of the forefoot, AP and 3/4 views.

Classification
None.

Treatment
Conservative treatment: Closed reduction by traction with a piece of gauze around the toe to obtain a better hold; for hallux luxation, use a splint for 1 week.
Surgical treatment: For dislocation that cannot be reduced; open reduction (remove plantar interposition) and the same treatment.

Duration
Injury takes 3 weeks to heal.
Duration of disability is 2 weeks.

Prognosis
Prognosis is good.

11.21 Toes fractures

Mechanism of injury
Direct force to the forefoot.

Clinical presentation
Local swelling. A hematoma occurs after a few days. Subungual hematoma is seen with a distal phalanx fracture.

Diagnostics
Physical examination: The affected toe is painful on palpation. Obvious hematoma.

X-ray examination: Only take x-rays of the forefoot to distinguish between intraarticular and extraarticular fractures.

Classification
- Shaft fracture
- Distal phalanx fracture
- Intraarticular/extraarticular fracture

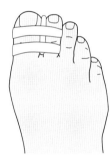

Fig 11-47   Method of taping a fractured toe.

Treatment
Conservative treatment: For all shaft fractures and distal phalanx fractures, toes are taped, leaving the affected toe free for 2 weeks. If the hallux is affected, a splint for 1 week is followed by a walking cast for 3 weeks.

Surgical treatment: For intraarticular fractures of the base of the phalanx (of the hallux) with displacement use open reduction and K-wires or screw fixation.

Duration
Injury takes 3–6 weeks to heal.
Duration of disability is 2–6 weeks.

Prognosis
Prognosis is good. If intraarticular fractures of the hallux cause problems with rolling the foot, special shoes or a metatarsal bar are indicated.

Part III

12 Complications of fracture healing

12.1 Delayed union

Delayed union happens when a fracture takes longer to heal than would normally be expected because of the location and type of fracture, associated soft-tissue injuries, and patient factors such as smoking.

Inadequate splinting, inexpert surgical technique, poor blood supply, and underlying infection can contribute to a delay in the fracture-healing process. In such cases, careful follow-up is essential and the therapeutic approach should be reassessed and adapted if necessary.

12.2 Nonunion (pseudarthrosis)

Pseudarthrosis is the failure of a fracture to unite within 9 months. The fracture ceases to show any evidence of healing and union will not occur with an intervention. Left untreated a true-false joint containing synovial fluid may develop between the bone ends. Symptomatic pseudarthrosis is always an indication for a change in the preexisting fracture treatment.

Etiology
- Unfavorable biomechanical conditions: usually inadequate stability
- Inadequate blood supply
- Anatomy of fracture: intracapsular femoral neck, scaphoid, or talus
- Trauma: high-energy injuries, open fractures, multifragmentary fractures with free-bone fragments
- Trauma of surgical intervention
- Infection
- Heavy smoking

Clinical presentation
Nonunion is characterized by painless abnormal mobility at the fracture site. There may be associated swelling and deformity, accompanied by loss of normal function.

Loss of muscle strength (upper extremities) and full weight-bearing ability (lower extremities) often occur.

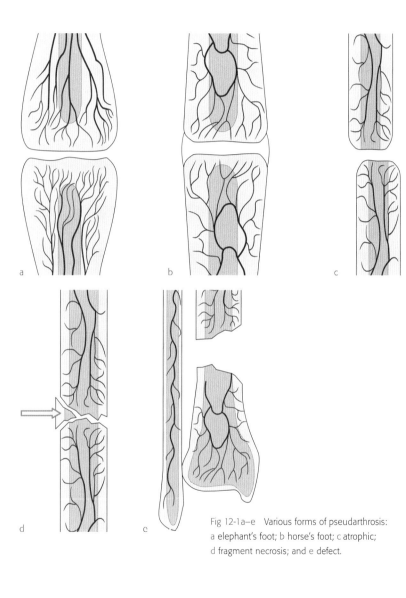

Fig 12-1a–e   Various forms of pseudarthrosis:
a elephant's foot; b horse's foot; c atrophic;
d fragment necrosis; and e defect.

Diagnostics
Physical examination: Dependent on localization.
X-ray examination: X-rays in two planes. If indicated, oblique views or CT scans.

Classification (Fig 12-1**)**

- Hypertrophic pseudarthrosis (etiology: mechanical) is characterized by widened, sclerotic extremities (elephant's or horse's foot) as a result of "nature" trying to bridge the fracture gap in an unstable injury. The bone ends are covered by fibrous cartilage and surrounded by a synovium-lined capsule, resembling a false joint.
- Atrophic pseudarthrosis (etiology: vascular); a result of an inadequate blood supply to the area; no bridging occurs, bone resorption is sometimes seen.
- Avulsion pseudarthrosis: muscle forces keep the bone end distracted.
- Defect pseudarthrosis: there is a bone defect.

Treatment
The choice of treatment depends on the type and localization of the pseudarthrosis. Symptoms can be limited, especially when upper extremities are affected. The movement in the false joint may rarely actually increase the function of the arm in which case stabilization results in a loss of function.

Surgical treatment: Stable fixation forms the basis of treatment for all types of pseudarthrosis. All implants that can be applied with compression are treatment options. Exceptions are the locked intramedullary nailing and tension band for specific indications.

Electromagnetic treatment: The osteoinductive effect of external or internal application of electromagnetic fields is under discussion. These stimulators are used in addition to surgery and cast immobilization. For this unproven method, long-term immobilization of the affected limb may be required.

Ultrasound treatment: The osteoinductive effect of low-frequency ultrasound applications has been established clinically and in animal studies. Results of this noninvasive treatment, in combination with external and internal immobilization, are promising. Ultrasound is given for 20 minutes once a day for fractures susceptible to delayed or nonunion.

Bone graft, bone graft substitutes, and recombinant bone morphogenetic protein (rhBMP): Due to their osteoconductive and osteoinductive properties, these have been used to promote healing especially in atrophic cases with or without a bone defect. Their value is still being assessed.

Treatment of hypertrophic pseudarthrosis: Rigid osteosynthesis soon leads to ossification of the cartilage and fibrous tissue in pseudarthrosis at any site. The chiseling away of small, vascularized callus fragments attached to the muscles (decortication) leads to a stimulating biological effect on bone healing. Additional autogenous bone grafting in this technique is not always necessary. Stable compression plating is a good technique and external fixation under compression is sometimes useful. Intramedullary nailing is a good treatment option for hypertrophic pseudarthrosis of the diaphysis of long bones. The medullary nail can be used to open the sclerotic bone ends and produce direct contact between the bone ends. The bone reamings or scrapings produced while inserting the nail constitute a biological stimulus. In a tibial pseudarthrosis, an intact fibula can prevent contact between the bone ends. Osteotomy of the fibula followed by weight-bearing ambulation in a short leg cast allows the tibial bone ends to come into contact, resulting in union of the tibia.

Treatment of atrophic pseudarthrosis: Characteristics of atrophic pseudarthroses are lack of callus, bone loss due to osteolysis, and formation of a synovial false joint. Rigid stabilization is needed but should be combined with decortication of the bone ends, removal of the synovial tissue, and autogenous bone grafting (iliac crests). The following types of bone grafts can be chosen: a solid tricortical iliac crest graft placed on the opposite side of the bone to the plate or as an interposition graft and a cancellous bone graft around the pseudarthrosis to ensure bone healing.

Treatment of avulsion pseudarthrosis: Examples are the lateral clavicle, epicondyles of the distal humerus, iliac crest, ischial tuberosity, greater trochanter, and tibial tuberosity. Lag screws ensure compression, and use of a tension band technique converts the tractive force of the muscles into compressive force.

Treatment of bone defect pseudarthrosis: A bone defect pseudarthrosis is by definition an atrophic pseudarthrosis with extensive bone loss. The above-mentioned treatment principles also apply to defects up to about 6 cm. Bone transport according to the Ilizarov method is the preferred treatment for larger defects, and such treatment is best performed in highly specialized units. For infected bone defect pseudarthrosis the treatment consists of external fixation for stabilization, multiple debridements, and free vascularized soft-tissue transfer if there is insufficient coverage of soft tissues. This is followed by (repeated) cancellous bone grafting or the Ilizarov method and occasionally free vascularized (fibular) bone grafting.

Treatment of pseudarthrosis of the femoral neck: For this rare form of pseudarthrosis, treatment needs to be individualized based on the patient's age and viability of the bone. In young patients, compression of the fracture ends can be achieved by an intertrochanteric valgization osteotomy according to the principles laid down by Pauwels. In the elderly, hip joint replacement is the preferred option.

Duration

The pseudarthrosis takes 2–3 months to heal when compression osteosynthesis and medullary nail fixation are used. For large defects, individual differences vary greatly with healing taking up to 1 year. Complications are the same for all forms of osteosynthesis. Reoperations because of complications (metal fatigue or supplementary cancellous bone grafting) are often needed.

The duration of disability is up to 2 months after consolidation of the pseudarthrosis. Most patients will have some residual disability even after solid bone union if treatment exceeds 1 year.

Prognosis

Modern techniques make it possible to achieve healing in all forms of pseudarthrosis. Recovery can be long. Therefore with a large infected bone defect or poor soft-tissue cover, amputation of a limb is sometimes an alternative allowing a speedy rehabilitation and return to work.

12.3 Malunion

Malunion is defined as the healing of bone in an abnormal position which with time can lead to problems and symptoms of a functional and/or cosmetic nature.

Etiology

With just a few exceptions, fractures usually consolidate without any form of treatment. In the absence of skilled supervision of alignment during healing, muscle contraction leads to shortening so that by definition healing results in a nonanatomical position (malunion). In this situation shortening is unavoidable, lateral displacement can be expected, and axial abnormalities and rotational deviations are common. The spontaneous correction that occurs in children should not be expected in adults.

Clinical presentation

The patient soon notices a shortening of the lower extremity; and/or angulation in the frontal or sagittal plane. Rotational problems sometimes go unnoticed. Patients and their families particularly focus on the esthetic aspects of malunion; overloading and pain play a less prominent role. The indication for corrective osteotomy is mainly determined by the clinical consequences of malunion in the long term.

Diagnostics

X-ray examination: Standard x-rays (for intraarticular malunion also oblique views) are generally adequate. It is important to compare the affected side with the other side because a preexisting deformity, such as valgus or varus deformity of the legs or anteversion of the femoral neck, could be corrected by the fracture. Shortening and rotational abnormalities are measured clinically. The same applies to the range of motion of the adjoining joints which could compensate for an existing deformity.

Classification

According to localization:

- Intraarticular
- Epiphyseal
- Metaphyseal
- Diaphyseal

According to malformation:
- Shortening/lengthening
- Valgus/varus
- Antecurvatum/recurvatum
- Rotation
- Combinations

Treatment of a short leg

No treatment is necessary for a limb-length discrepancy of up to 2 cm, while shoe correction provides an adequate effect for a discrepancy up to 2.5 cm. If the discrepancy is more than 2.5 cm surgical treatment is indicated, tailored to the needs and wishes of the patient. If there are no axial abnormalities, shortening of the nonaffected limb by osteotomy is advisable because few complications occur with this treatment. Intertrochanteric shortening of the femur is associated with least complications. Bone lengthening using the Ilizarov method is an alternative. This treatment requires endurance from the patient and has a high complication rate especially in the femur.

Treatment of an intraarticular abnormality: The joint anatomy is restored by means of osteotomy and stable osteosynthesis, followed by functional follow-up treatment.

Treatment of an epiphyseal or metaphyseal abnormality: Correction of the deformity and fixation with a plate and screws or external fixation. An open- or closed-wedge technique can be chosen, depending on the difference in length, type of deformity, and presence of ligament instability.

Treatment of a diaphyseal abnormality: The mid point of the hip, knee, and ankle should form one straight line. Curves in between these points are not significant, as long as the knee and ankle are loaded horizontally. The correction of a diaphyseal abnormality is preferably performed at the level of the metaphysis because an osteotomy heals more rapidly at that location. Plates and screws are implants of choice for correction of metaphyseal and intraarticular malunions. Stable fixation and functional follow-up treatment after an osteotomy are more important than for the treatment of new fractures. Compression osteotomy with external fixation is possible if transfixation pins do not irritate the tendons and muscles too much, and the risk of joint infection is minimal (proximal and distal tibia). For corrections at the diaphyseal level, the medullary nail is the ideal implant.

Duration

An osteotomy heals within 6–8 weeks. Lengthening and/or callus distraction progresses at an average of 0.5–1 mm daily. Pseudarthroses can occur when lengthening procedures are used, while these complications are rare with other osteotomies.

Long-term disability often occurs as a result of malunion. Work can sometimes be resumed about 4 months after osteotomy, except after a lengthening procedure.

Prognosis

An osteotomy of a posttraumatic deformity that is optimally planned and performed technically correctly restores normal biomechanics and prevents secondary problems.

13 Contractures and chronic ligament instability

13   Contractures and chronic ligament instability

13.1   Contractures

A contracture is a loss of range of movement in a joint. It can be caused by tightening of soft tissues around a joint or by changes within the joint itself—both bony and soft tissue. The following types are distinguished:

A flexion contracture: tightening in flexion when the joint cannot be fully extended.

An extension contracture: tightening in extension when the joint cannot be fully flexed.

■ A contracture refers only to a passive range of motion. If there is a difference between active and passive mobility, this is known as a deficit. For example, there is an extension deficit if the knee can be extended further passively than actively.

Classification
Classification is based on the underlying cause.

Intraarticular:
- Adhesions due to long-term immobilization (eg, finger joints, wrist, knee)
- Secondary (posttraumatic) arthrosis (after fracture of joint)
- Avascular necrosis
- Large joint effusion or hemarthrosis

Periarticular:
- Posttraumatic dystrophy of muscle, tendon, and capsule
- Malunion of a fracture close to a joint
- Periarticular ossifications

Extraarticular:
- Muscle adhesions at the site of the fracture
- Fibrosis of the muscles, eg, after compartment syndrome
- Hypertonia or spasticity of the muscles
- Scarring of skin

Treatment

Conservative treatment: Prevention is better than cure. Contractures can be prevented through awareness of possible causes.

Treatment is difficult, painful, and lengthy. Contractures occurring after the treatment of fractures often recover spontaneously, therefore patience is advisable. Good pain management is important, as well as active exercises. Do not concentrate only on improving the range of motion passively. An intraarticular injection of a local anesthetic sometimes breaks the pain spiral.

Surgical treatment: Arthrotomy with resection of obstructing callus and ossifications and the division of adhesions. Corrective periarticular osteotomy can be used to "reposition" the joint to obtain a better functional range of motion.

■ These operations require extensive experience from the surgeon and careful patient selection; results are unpredictable and rehabilitation programs are prolonged.

13.2 Chronic ligament instability

Acute injuries of the ligaments associated with instability are common in the ankle, knee, and thumb. Chronic ligament instability is relatively rare, except in the shoulder, wrist, knee, and ankle.

Recurrent and habitual shoulder dislocation/instability

Recurrent shoulder dislocation is a frequently repeated dislocation of the shoulder joint that occurs without severe force after an initial traumatic dislocation.

Habitual shoulder dislocation is a frequent dislocation of the shoulder occurring during normal movement without an initial traumatic dislocation.

Etiology, pathogenesis, pathophysiology

The etiology and pathogenesis of habitual shoulder dislocation are not yet fully understood.

Predisposing factors are:
■ Anomalies in the capsuloligamentous apparatus
■ Changes in the collagen linkages or composition of the capsule
■ Dysplasic glenoid
■ Increased anteversion of the glenoid, reduced retrotorsion of the humeral head

- Congenital weakness of the connective tissue (Ehlers-Danlos syndrome, Marfan syndrome)
- Muscular degeneration

The first dislocation normally occurs anteriorly and inferiorly in young patients without adequate traumatic cause (Fig 13-1).

The resulting instability is often multidirectional and seldom causes much pain.

The younger the patient is when the first traumatic shoulder dislocation occurs the greater the risk of recurrence. For patients younger than 25 years, the risk is nearly 90%; whereas for those older than 65 years, it is less than 10%. Arthroscopy for first dislocations is strongly recommended for patients younger than 25 years.

A common cause of recurrent shoulder dislocation is an avulsion of the anteroinferior labrum off the glenoid rim (Bankart injury) which results in loss of function in the inferior and medial glenohumeral ligaments. In addition, the anteroinferior capsule is stretched with posterolateral displacement of the humeral head; an impression fracture of the humeral head can occur as a result of the initial dislocation (Hill-Sachs lesion). This bony defect may also contribute to recurrent dislocation.

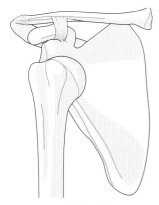

Fig 13-1 Anterior shoulder dislocation.

Gerber classification of instability:

Type I: Chronically locked dislocation
Type II: Unidirectional instability with no hyperlaxity
Type III: Unidirectional instability with multidirectional hyperlaxity
Type IV: Multidirectional instability with no hyperlaxity
Type V: Multidirectional instability with multidirectional hyperlaxity
Type VI: Voluntary instability

Accompanying injuries: Hill-Sachs defect, bony Bankart lesion, rotator cuff rupture, ACJ dislocation, clavicular fracture, tuberculum majus fracture, or glenoid fracture.

Clinical diagnostic procedures

Visual inspection—evaluation of:

- Appearance of both shoulders (asymmetry)
- Adaptive posture
- Musculature
- Swelling

Palpation—evaluation of:

- Fluid
- Tenderness
- Crepitation

Specific function and pain tests:

- Mobility test (active and passive, rotation mobility in 0° and 90° abduction)
- Apprehension test
- Drawer test
- Sulcus sign
- Relocation test
- Jerk test
- Fulcrum test
- Drop arm sign

Diagnostic procedures:

- X-ray of the shoulder with two views

Further tests useful in individual cases:

- Ultrasound (primarily to rule out a rotator cuff lesion)
- Special x-ray projections, eg, Velpeau view (position of the humeral head relative to the glenoid), ventrodorsal view with 60° internal rotation (Hill-Sachs), glenoid rim view
- Magnetic resonance imaging (MRI)

Treatment of recurrent dislocation

Reduction using axial and lateral traction (Arlt, Matsen) under the influence of analgesics or anesthetics.

Surgical treatment: Refixation of the labral lesion if present (also known as a Bankart injury) to the anterior glenoid. This operation can be performed either as an open surgery or by arthroscopy. The open method results in fewer recurrences. Operations in which a rotating osteotomy is used to turn a posterolateral defect of the humeral head (also known as Hill-Sachs injury) more laterally are performed less frequently, despite reported good results.

Wrist

Dorsal intercalated segment instability (DISI), often linked to scapholunate dissociation, is usually the result of an injury to the scapholunar ligament. This rupture is often associated with a fracture of the wrist but also occurs in isolation. Volar intercalated segment instability (VISI) is the result of an injury of the lunatotriquetral ligament. Both forms of intercarpal instability are rare.

Diagnosis			
	Grade I	**Grade II**	**Grade III**
Watson test	Positive	Positive	Positive
Plain x-ray	Negative	Negative	Positive
Stress x-ray	Negative	Positive	
Dynamic x-ray	Negative	Positive	
Arthrography	Positive	Positive	Positive
Arthroscopy	Positive	Positive	Positive

Table 13-1   Scapholunate ligament injury.

Classification:

- Grade I: partial rupture in the middle membranous section with no displacement of the scaphoid and lunate
- Grade II: complete rupture with dynamic instability of the scaphoid
- Grade III: complete rupture with static instability matching the visible criteria for SL-Dissociation with the scaphoid in flexion and lunate in extension (DISI position) (Fig 13-2)

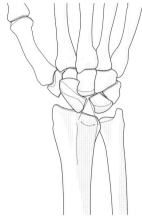

Fig 13-2   Wrist showing widening of the joint space as sign of rupture of scapholunate ligament.

Treatment of an acute injury (< 6 weeks after injury)

■ Grade I: cast immobilization for 4–6 weeks

■ Grades II and III: surgical repair, stabilization with K-wires and immobilization with cast for 8 weeks

Treatment of a chronic injury (> 6 weeks from injury)

■ Ligament reconstruction: using flexor carpi radialis (Brunelli procedure)

■ Dorsal capsulodesis (Blatt procedure) rarely used nowadays

■ Limited carpal fusion (particularly if symptomatic local arthrosis)

Mayo Classification for wrist instability

CID (carpal instability dissociative): ligaments between bones in the same carpal row are injured

CIND (carpal instability nondissociative): ligaments between bones in different carpal rows are injured

CIC (carpal instability complex): a combination of CID and CIND exist

CIA (carpal instability adaptive): there is no ligament injury, but the bones assume an abnormal position because of alteration in their shape or platform (eg, distal radius malunion)

Thumb

Chronic instability is most common as the result of an undetected injury to the ulnar collateral ligament of the metacarpophalangeal joint of the thumb.

Distribution:

1. Partial tear
2. Complete rupture
3. Bony avulsion of the collateral ligament apparatus

Operative treatment: Tendon plasty with a tendon graft produces the best improvement in stability, but is associated with some loss in flexion. In acute cases repair of the ruptured ligament is often possible.

Knee

The stability of the knee is mainly determined by the anterior cruciate ligament (ACL) and collateral ligaments. Acute rupture of ACL is common. It cannot repair itself, probably because of poor blood supply to this area ("Le Pivot central ne cicatrise jamais"). The consequences of an injury to the ACL can vary from no symptoms to disabling instability. It is not known whether a chronic ACL lesion is linked to a high risk of arthrosis.

Clinical tests of anterior instability	
Lachman test (Anterior tibia translation in comparison with uninvolved side) (Fig 13-3a)	**Pivot shift test** (Fig 13-3b–d)
Grade I (+): Translation 3–5 mm, firm end point, ACL intact	**Grade I:** only demonstrable in internal rotation
Grade II (++): Translation 6–10 mm, end point softened, ACL stretched	**Grade II:** demonstrable in neutral position
Grade III (+++): Translation >10 mm, soft/nonexistent end point, ACL deficient	**Grade III:** demonstrable in external rotation

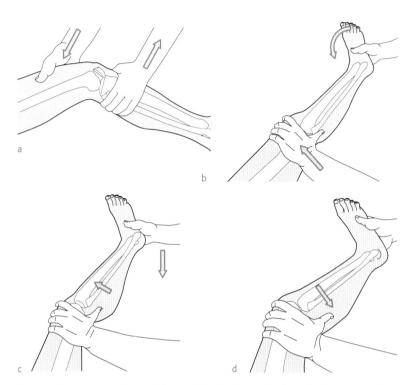

Fig 13-3a–d Tests for anterior instability: a Pulling the tibia anteriorly results in anterior translation of the tibia on the femur. b Internal rotation of the foot with gentle anterior pressure on the
fibular head subluxes lateral side of proximal tibia anteriorally. c Flexion of knee. d With further
flexion ilio-tibial band caused subluxation to reduce suddenly—pivot shift.

Treatment

Conservative treatment: Intensive exercises to increase muscle strength
and proprioception; use a brace during exercise and sometimes also for other
activities.

Surgical treatment: Secondary reconstruction is often performed to treat
chronic injuries of ACL. The treatment of choice is reconstruction with a graft
either harvested from the patient's patellar tendon (bone–tendon–bone graft)
or created from the semitendinosus tendon using the double or quadruple
stranded method. Reconstruction with a synthetic prosthesis is no longer performed.

Chronic symptoms arising from instability to injury to the posterior cruciate ligament are rare. Pain is more likely to occur than instability problems (more disability than instability). Reconstruction with bone–tendon–bone graft or semitendinosus ligament is possible but difficult.

Follow-up treatment: A brace for 4–6 weeks or full functional treatment with progressive weight bearing using crutches. Intensive muscle-strengthening exercises.

Duration: Injury takes 4–6 weeks to heal. The duration of disability is mainly dependent on the patient's profession and the load to the knee, 6 weeks minimum. Regular sporting activities can be resumed after 4–6 months, but contact sport (eg, football, handball, or judo) only after 1 year.

Ankle

When chronic instability of the ankle joint is caused by injuries to the lateral ligaments, it can be treated well and reliably by surgery if conservative treatment fails. The diagnosis of chronic anterolateral rotary instability (ALRI) should always be considered for patients with chronic instability of the ankle joint. Many diagnostic methods have been reported, but invasive techniques are being used less frequently.

Typical complaints

Unsteady gait on uneven ground, inability to take part in sporting activities, or fear of repeated twisting of the ankle.

Clinical complaints

Synovitic irritation in the upper ankle joint, chronic tendovaginitis, painful contracture, or atrophy of the peroneal muscles.

Diagnostics of ALRI

Radiological tests: Anterior drawer (Figs 13-4a, 13-5) and talar tilt stress x-ray (Fig 13-6) on two planes (Figs 13-4b, 13-7) using local anesthesia. Compare with the uninjured side. Ultrasound examination of the ankle joint is better.

Standardized clinical evaluation: Demonstrable anterior drawer sign and lateral tilt of the talus with the foot in plantar flexion, instability in the subtalar joint when subjected to varus stress with the foot in dorsiflexion.

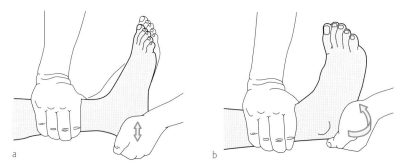

Fig 13-4a–b a Anterior drawer test; b talar tilt test.

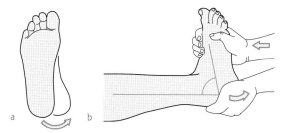

Fig 13-5a–b a Test of subtalar movement with the foot in dorsi-flexion; b movements of calcaneocuboid joint under varus stress of the hindfoot.

Clinical	X-ray		Sonography
TT and AD	TT°	AD, mm	ADS (mm) print
1+	5–9	5–7	3–4
2+	10–15	8–10	5–6
3+	16–30	>10	>7

Table 13-2 Criteria of anterolateral rotary instability in the upper ankle joint. TT indicates talus tilt; AD, anterior drawer; and ADS, anterior drawer observed with sonography.

Chronic ALRI of ankle joint: This is a result of injuries to the lateral ligaments without treatment or multiple supination traumas.

Treatment
Surgical stabilization of lateral collateral ligaments usually using the tendon of peroneus brevis (Watson-Jones plasty).

Other instabilities are the uncommon calcaneocuboid instability (Fig 13-5a–b) and combined upper/lower ankle joint instability. These are treated operatively.

Follow-up treatment: Upper leg cast for 8–10 days, then proprioceptive reflex training. In addition, a shoe with a 0.5 cm built-up rim can be recommended for 6 months.

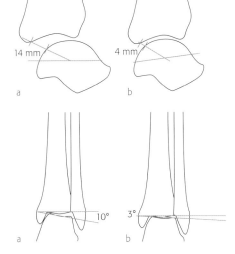

Fig 13-6a–b   Measurement anterior drawer test.

Fig 13-7a–b   Radiographic measuring of talar tilt test.

14 Compartment syndrome and posttraumatic dystrophy

14   Compartment syndrome and posttraumatic dystrophy

14.1   Compartment syndrome

Compartment syndrome is a condition in which the blood circulation and the function of the (neuromuscular) tissue in a confined space (compartment) are compromised because of an increased pressure within that space. Irreversible loss of function can result.

Conditions
Two conditions exist for compartment syndrome to occur:
- Presence of a compartment containing neuromuscular tissue
- A cause for a rise in pressure within that compartment

Compartment syndrome can occur in almost every muscle or muscle group in the body.

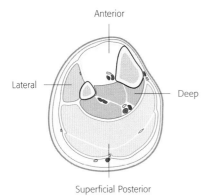

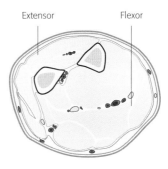

Fig 14-1   Cross-section of the lower leg showing four different compartments.

Fig 14-2   Cross-section of the forearm showing different compartments.

Causes

A reduction in the volume of the compartment or an increase in its content can lead to compartment syndrome.

Reduction in the volume of the compartment can be caused by:
- A bandage or plaster cast that is too tight
- Closure of a fascial defect
- Thermal injury

An increase in the contents of the compartment can be caused by:
Edema:
- Postischemic
- Patient's own body weight after a drug overdose
- Thermal injuries
- After exercise
- Compromised venous return
- Paravascular injection
- Poison (snakebite)

Bleeding:
- Clotting disorder (congenital or drug induced)
- Vascular injuries

Combination of edema and bleeding:
- Fracture or osteotomy
- Soft-tissue injuries

Clinical presentation

Clinical signs and symptoms of acute compartment syndrome are:
- Pain (continuous and disproportional)
- Swollen, tender compartment
- Pain on passively stretching muscles in the affected compartment
- Neurological deficit (sensory)
- Muscle weakness

  - The symptoms are arranged in chronological order. The more symptoms are present, the more serious the situation. Neurological deficit and muscle weakness are later signs. Treatment should be initiated before these signs occur.

■ Arterial pulses are present, unless arterial injuries are the cause of the compartment syndrome. Absence of peripheral pulses should not be relied on to diagnose compartment syndrome.

Diagnostics

Diagnosis of a compartment syndrome is based on clinical signs:

- Soft-tissue injuries
- Disproportionate pain
- Pain on passive stretching of muscle
- A tense compartment
- Muscle weakness
- The presence of a fracture, including stress fractures and osteotomies

Causes of compartment syndrome can include:

- Cellulitis
- Osteomyelitis
- Tenosynovitis
- Deep vein thrombosis
- Acute vascular occlusion and reperfusion injury following arterial reconstruction

The symptom complex may not present fully due to patient-related factors:

- Noncooperative patient
- Coma
- A child
- Preexisting peripheral neurological disorder
- Use of local anesthetic for pain relief (including epidurals)

If in doubt, intracompartmental pressure measurement is the only way to reach a definite diagnosis. When the tissue pressure is higher than 30 mm Hg, decompression should be performed. The difference between diastolic blood pressure and tissue pressure may also be used (<30 mm Hg is an indication for immediate decompression).

Other measuring method (creatine kinase, myoglobinuria, electromyogram, laser Doppler, muscle Po2, MRI, CT scan, or echography) only provide indirect indications of the possibility of compartment syndrome, and only after irreversible damage has occurred. If a measuring device is not available, then the diagnosis and management are based on clinical findings.

Treatment

The treatment of acute compartment syndrome consists of decompression:

- Remove the tight bandage or plaster cast
- Escharotomy (decompression of the skin)—in cases of burns
- Fasciotomy
- Epimysiotomy (decompression of the connective tissue between muscles and fascia)

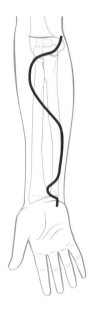

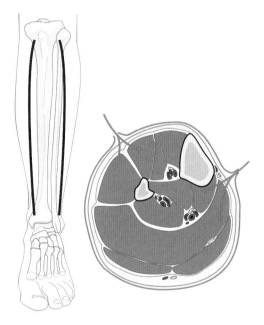

Fig 14-3   Palmar incision for decompression of the forearm.

Fig 14-4   Lateral and medial incisions for decompression of all four compartments of the lower leg.

■ As there is a linear relationship between duration of the raised pressure and risk of irreversible damage, it is important to achieve decompression as soon as possible.

■ Fasciotomy must be performed as an "open" procedure, whereby all affected compartments are completely exposed without causing any additional neurovascular damage. Wounds should remain open until swelling has resolved sufficiently. Fasciotomy is never performed as a closed procedure.

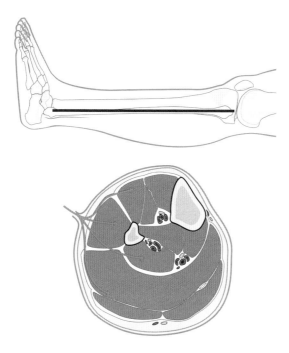

Fig 14-5   Lateral incision for decompression of all four compartments of the lower leg.

Prevention

Prevention of acute compartment syndrome:

- Do not apply bandages too tightly
- For new injuries use a splint or a fully split circular cast
- Instruct the patient and family/friends to look out for signs and symptoms and to immediately seek help and treatment if necessary
- Prevent hypotension
- Do not elevate the limb too high
- Restrict traction to the limb
- Perform a prophylactic fasciotomy after vascular reconstructions

  - Consequences of missing a diagnosis of compartment syndrome and thus delaying or failing to start treatment can lead to serious disability contracture formation or even require amputation.

14.2   Posttraumatic dystrophy

Posttraumatic dystrophy (PTD) is a symptom complex in which at least three of the following symptoms exist after trauma:

- Inexplicable, diffuse pain
- A difference in skin color and/or temperature compared with the other limb
- Diffuse edema
- Restriction in the range of motion of (small) joints
- Occurrence or deterioration of these symptoms when the affected limb is used
- The area where symptoms have occurred is more extensive than the originally affected area and includes at least the periphery of the limb and the injury site

In 90% of cases, there is a history of evident injury (trauma or surgical intervention). PTD is more common in the upper extremities than the lower extremities and more often seen in women than men.

Dystrophy should be considered in all patients complaining of pain that is not proportional to the nature of the traumatic injury; it is essential to examine the patient for physical signs of PTD. By diagnosing PTD early and starting treatment at once, the chance that the symptom complex will resolve is highest.

Treatment

There is no consensus regarding the pathogenesis of PTD. Theories include inactivity, a psychogenic cause, injury to the sympathetic nervous system, and an abnormal inflammatory reaction. Consensus is, however, increasingly being reached with treatment.

Treatment includes numerous measures which focus on improving oxygenation at the cellular level so that the initial increase in the blood supply to the limb normalizes. In this way, pain gradually subsides and the restriction in range of motion is eased. Complete recovery may not occur; in such cases chronic pain syndrome remains with severe loss of function. Although there is a risk that PTD will recur in patients, surgical interventions are allowed, as long as they are indicated; intervention may even contribute to a reduction or recovery of PTD.

Treatment consists of:
- Gradually increasing exercise therapy as pain permits, with mobilization of peripheral joints
- Cryotherapy
- Empirically tested medication (DMSO cream or spray, mannitol, prednisolone, vitamin C, and so on)
- Nonsteroidal antiinflammatory drugs (NSAIDs) and other analgesics
- Neuromedications, ie, amytriptaline, pregabalin, and gabapentin
- If present: trigger point treatment
- In the cold phase—blocking of the sympathetic nerve (stellate blocks, lumbar sympathectomy)

With chronic "cold dystrophy" (less pain, more loss of function) peripheral vasodilatation by means of medication or sympathectomy can be useful. Accompanying pain in the shoulder, which is seen in 20% of patients with PTD of the upper extremities, responds well to infiltration with corticosteroids and a local anesthetic.

All those treating patients with traumatic injuries should be well informed of the above-mentioned symptom complex. The relatively high frequency (8%) of PTD in trauma patients justifies an active approach. At the slightest suspicion of PTD the diagnosis should be made accurately, followed by early treatment.

Due to the slow recovery and uncertainty regarding the extent to which disabling symptoms will resolve, the treatment and management of patients with PTD should be performed with great care. Patients and their caregivers should be informed of the uncertain prognosis.

15 Osteoporosis

15.1 Introduction

Osteoporosis has been defined by the World Health Organization as "A systemic skeletal disease characterized by low bone mass and microarchitectural deterioration with a consequent increase in bone fragility with susceptibility to fracture."

15.2 Epidemiology

Osteoporosis is described as the silent epidemic. People affected by the disease usually have no symptoms until a fracture occurs. It is estimated that one in three women and one in 12 men older than 50 years worldwide have osteoporosis. The number of people older than 80 years will triple in the next 40 years and there will be a twofold to fourfold increase in the number of fragility fracture occurring worldwide in the next 30 years. In Europe the number of fragility fractures will increase from 4 million to 6.7 million cases per year; in Asia it will reach 32.5 million cases per year by 2050.

Currently in the United States more than 250,000 hip fractures per year are caused by osteoporosis. A 50-year-old white woman has a 17.5% lifetime risk of a fracture of the proximal femur. The incidence of hip fractures increases each decade from the sixth to the ninth in both men and women.

Vertebral fractures occur in between 35% and 50% of all women older than 60 years. Up to two-thirds of these are unrecognized and the annual incidence in the United States may exceed 700,000 cases annually.

The costs of treating these fractures will soar from $17.5 billion to $45 billion within 10 years in the United States alone.

15.3 Pathogenesis

The underlying mechanism in all osteoporosis cases is an imbalance between the normal bone absorption and formation that occur as part of normal bone turnover. Changes happen in the cortical bone where a decreased thickness of the cortices is accompanied by an increase in the bone diameter (Fig 15-1). The microstructure of the cortices also changes with increased Haversian canal areas which cause increased weakness and a predisposition to low-energy fractures (Fig 15-2). The cancellous bone also changes—the trabeculae become less with fewer, often broken interconnections (Fig 15-3).

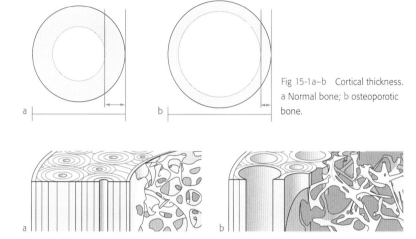

Fig 15-1a–b   Cortical thickness. a Normal bone; b osteoporotic bone.

Fig 15-2a–b   a Normal bone; b increased Haversian canal areas in osteoporotic bone.

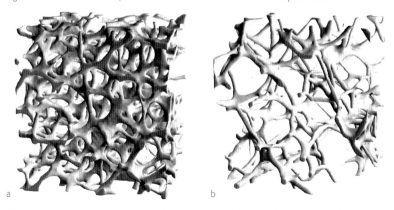

Fig 15-3a–b   a Young, normal lumbar spine; b osteoporotic lumbar spine. (Courtesy of Ralph Müller Swiss Federal Institute of Technology, Zürich).

Bone mass increases during growth and reaches a peak between 30 and 40 years. The peak bone mass achieved by any patient is related to the nutritional intake as well as the amount of physical activity undertaken. Weight-bearing exercise encourages an increase in bone mass and a sedentary lifestyle reduces this occurrence. After 40 years there is a natural reduction in bone mass that can be reduced but not neutralized by physical activity and changes in lifestyle—senile osteoporosis.

An inadequate peak bone mass, excessive bone resorption, and inadequate formation of new bone during remodeling are the three main mechanisms by which osteoporosis develops. A lack of estrogen increases bone resorption and is the most important factor in the development of postmenopausal osteoporosis in women.

15.4   Risk factors

Not modifiable:
- Advancing age
- Estrogen deficiency
- Testosterone deficiency
- Strong family history

Modifiable:
- Vitamin D deficiency
- Smoking
- Excess alcohol consumption
- Low body mass index
- Malnutrition especially low calcium intake
- Physical inactivity
- Excess consumption of carbonated drinks

Diseases:
- Immobilization, eg, disuse osteoporosis with cast immobilization
- Endocrine disorders, especially Cushing's syndrome, hyperparathyroidism, thyrotoxicosis, and adrenal insufficiency
- Malnutrition including medical causes, eg, postmastectomy
- Renal insufficiency
- Autoimmune diseases, eg, rheumatoid arthritis and systemic lupus erythematosis

Medications
- Steroids
- Phenytoin and some barbiturates
- Methotrexate
- Long-term lithium therapy

15.5   Diagnosis

Osteoporosis is diagnosed by measuring the bone mineral density (BMD). The most common method is the use of dual energy x-ray absorptiometry (DEXA).

Osteoporosis is diagnosed when the bone mineral density is less than or equal to 2.5 standard deviations below that of the average young adult. This is known as the "T-score":

> T-score = -1.0 or more is normal
> T-score between -1.0 and -2.5 is osteopenia
> T-score -2.5 or below is osteoporosis

Any woman patient older than 70 years with an insufficiency fracture can be assumed to have osteoporosis.

Clinical presentation
Most patients present first with a fracture. Fracture occur following minimal or even no trauma—a pathological fracture. The most common presenting fractures are of the distal radius, proximal femur, proximal humerus, and pubic rami. Spontaneous fractures of the vertebral bodies are also common with many of the fractures being pain free. For pain-free patients presentation is caused by loss of height or the development of a deformity.

15.6 Treatment

Drug therapy can significantly reduce the risk of a second osteoporotic fracture occurring in patients whose presentation came about as a result of a fracture. Drugs can also reduce the risk of a first fracture in those patients whose osteoporosis was diagnosed as a result of screening. Alendronate reduces the risk of recurrent fracture after vertebral fractures by 47%. Similar risk reduction is seen with the use of zoledronic acid. Antiresoptives reduce the risk of recurrent hip fractures by 26% in elderly patients.

Despite clear evidence that treating osteoporotic patients has benefits, the rates of evaluation of osteoporosis and treatment of osteoporotic patients following fracture remains disappointingly low.

The orthopaedic treatment of these patients focuses on techniques which allow rapid return to function. In lower extremity injuries the priority is a procedure that will allow the patient to get out of bed and mobilize rapidly. Prolonged period of bed rest results in a high level of complications including bed sores, hypostatic pneumonia, and thromboembolic disease. Implants which allow early weight bearing, such as intramedullary nails (Fig 15-4) greatly facilitate mobilization since the elderly have insufficient strength to mobilize partial or nonweight bearing. Upper limb injuries also demand rapid return of function and the development of newer plating systems suitable for osteoporotic bone has significantly changed treatment regimen.

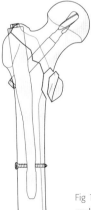

Fig 15-4   Unstable pertrochanteric femoral fracture treated with cephalomedullary device.

Vertebral fractures can now be treated by minimally invasive techniques such as kyphoplasty.

15.7 Prognosis

Osteoporotic patients who present with a fracture have two sets of problems:
1. Most of these patients are elderly and have several significant comorbidities. These comorbidities require comanagement by the medical team with close cooperation between orthopaedic surgeons, geriatricians, and anesthetists. The 30-day mortality for a proximal femoral fracture varies between 8% and 15%. Up to 20% of patients are readmitted within 30 days of discharge. Perioperative mortality and morbidity can be dramatically reduced by comanagement of these patients by the relevant specialities and many protocols have been designed to facilitate initial care.
2. Osteoporotic bone has profoundly different biomechanical characteristics compared with normal bone. Certain internal fixation techniques and implants fail when used in osteoporotic patients because of a weak hold in the bone. Implants which allow collapse of the fracture are favored.

The combination of these problems results in a poor prognosis for many patients. Approximately 70% of patients presenting with a proximal femoral fracture were able to undertake basic activities of daily living. This figure reduces to 40% 1 year after fracture. Some 64% of patients may require nursing home care within 1 year of hip fracture.

Successful management of patients with osteoporotic bone fracture is a team effort. Anesthesists provide expertise in evaluation and may frequently have to adapt techniques to deal with patients who would be refused elective surgery on health grounds. Geriatricians provide help with assessment, postoperative medical care, and rehabilitation. The orthopaedic surgeon provides expertise on fracture management and may in turn have to adapt his or her technique to deal with the problems of fixation in osteoporotic bone.

16 Documentation

16 Documentation

16.1 Introduction

Trauma is extremely prevalent in contemporary society. It causes lost time from work and school as well as impacting costs to the individual and the community. Clinical evaluation upon hospital admission can save lives and prevents worsening of diagnosed injuries.

Protocols have been established to perform a systematic evaluation that assesses and manages life-threatening injuries. Once a patient is more stable, other disabling injuries are investigated and properly managed.

16.2 Objective and implications

Trauma management is a dynamic situation which involves a multidisciplinary approach; thus, documentation is paramount. Documenting every step of diagnosis and treatment makes the information available to every member of the health care team, and offers parameters for clinical judgment. It is vital in case of legal inquiries. Good documentation provides data for research, treatment comparison, and quality control.

Case history

A history of the injury is recorded to gain insight into the cause of trauma, with focus on injury-related energy and contamination.

Anatomical and functional disabilities are documented by clinical and x-ray examinations. Photographs, if necessary with a mobile phone, are taken to document soft-tissue conditions at admission and after surgical debridements. This is especially important in cases of mangled extremities to support decisions made as limb salvage or amputation.

Orthopaedic evaluation

Orthopaedic evaluation of polytrauma patients involves a head-to-toe detailed physical examination. The time of injury and the interval until medical assistance arrived are important, since delay in treatment can have critical outcome. For example, open fractures managed within 6 hours of a trauma episode have different grades of contamination compared with similar fractures with greater time of exposure.

Medical history

Earlier disorders or treatments should be investigated and documented. Patients with previous orthopaedic surgeries are a challenge to manage, since they can present with broken or deformed implants together with their new injuries.

As life expectancy is increasing, the elderly are common among trauma patients. They usually present with osteoporotic bone fractures together with comorbidities, such as diabetes mellitus, cardiac insufficiency, cancer, or dementia. Any of these conditions should be assessed for a better understanding of the case; thus, helping to devise an efficient treatment plan.

X-ray assessment

X-ray assessment is essential for interpreting the magnitude of trauma event and planning the orthopaedic approach. X-rays should be of good quality. X-rays that do not depict the whole bone segment, and those done with poor techniques are not acceptable.

Orthopaedic surgeons in charge of trauma management should be critical when accepting images that could prevent an accurate diagnosis. Ipsilateral neck and diaphyseal femoral fractures are frequently missed because of incomplete x-rays that do not depict the whole femur.

Computed tomography (CT) enables whole body scans within a few minutes. If available, a CT scan is valuable especially for depicting spine and articular injuries.

Injury Severity Score

Trauma scores take into account hemodynamic status and the overall injury extension—cavities, organs, and systems. These scores are not so precise as to determine outcomes but can guide some medical decisions. Injury Severity Score (ISS) gives a classification of trauma magnitudes.

The ISS is calculated using a simple formula based on the severity of the separate injuries to six organ systems: central nervous system, thorax, abdomen, limbs, soft tissues, and circulation. Overall, ISS equals or higher than 40 is an indication for damage-control orthopaedics instead of early total care of fractures.

Documentation for victims of abuse

A detailed description of injuries is required for victims of violence and abuse. Complete assessment and documentation including x-rays and photographic images and a descriptive report is the best evidence for legal purposes.

International Classification of Diseases

Diagnostics should be coded according to the International Classification of Diseases (ICD 10). AO provides an alphanumeric classification for bone and soft-tissue injuries. Classification is useful if universally accepted and easy to understand. Its value is also to guide treatment and to estimate outcomes.

Medical intervention

Describe all medical intervention fully, ie, drug administration (doses and intervals), venous accesses, emergency procedures (splints, skeletal traction), and surgical procedures (time since trauma episode, duration, technique, implant selection, and image intensifier control data).

Polytrauma patients often undergo multiple interventions. At the end of treatment, results are analyzed interpreting all recorded data. This procedure reinforces some technical approaches and identifies failed protocols that should be revised.

During surgical procedures all intermediary images obtained by the image intensifier should be stored. This helps to understand end results, documenting every surgical step, and any complications.

Complications can be related to injury or to treatment. They should be documented as well as the methods used to manage them.

Assessing end results

End results are documented on clinical reports and imaging. Fracture healing is a biological process best followed up by x-rays analyses. X-rays should have the same exposure, avoiding misinterpretations.

All x-rays are stored to compare the evolution of fracture healing. Any orthopaedic treatment is to restore anatomy and function of an injured area. Limb function restoration involves reestablishment of length, rotation, and alignment. Articular restoration concerns anatomical reduction and restitution of complete range of motion.

16.3 Neutral-0-method

Evaluation of articular function is essential for documenting partial or complete disabilities because of trauma or treatment. The neutral-0-method offers the opportunity to register the range of motion of the affected joint or the adjoining joints clearly and unambiguously.

Anatomical positioning

The neutral-0-method is based on the basic anatomical position from which all measurements are taken. This position involves the patient standing upright, arms hanging by the sides with thumbs pointing forward. The functional longitudinal axes of the feet are parallel and separated by a space equal to the distance between the hips. The gaze is directed forward and horizontally. This position is the starting point for each measurement; the position of each joint is 0° (Fig 16-1). Normal values are equivalent to the average range of joint movement in healthy adults. However, comparison of each pair of joints is essential when defining abnormal findings.

Three numbers define every joint movement: the two ends of the range movement and the 0-position. If the 0-position is passed, the zero is always located between the two measured end-position values. The values of

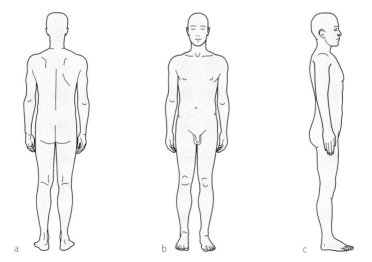

a   b   c

Fig 16-1a–c   Starting point with neutral-0 position of the joints.

120°/0°/5° registered during a knee examination mean that this joint has a flexion range of 120° and an extension range of 5°.

Joint contractures can also be described. In these cases, if neutral position is not attained the numeral 0 is inserted either in front of or behind the two measured readings. With the knee joint as a model, values of 120°/40°/0° mean 80° range of flexion or a 40° flexion contracture in the knee joint. Joint movements should be measured actively and passively. Range of movement for every joint can be assessed and recorded with this method (Figs 16-2, 16-3, 16-4, 16-5, 16-6, 16-7).

Quality control
Length and girth measurements are performed in the normal anatomical position and should, if possible, be compared with the opposite side. Reference bony landmarks are used to measure the length. Different observer should be able to reproducibly locate these landmarks. In the lower limb, anterosuperior iliac spine and medial malleolus are usually taken to estimate lower limb length.

Girth measurements are performed at defined points, usually at whole number intervals from bony landmarks (eg, circumference of thigh 12 cm above superior pole of patella).

Medicolegal inquiries
Ability to walk and to return to functional capabilities existing before an injury is an important parameter to judge the impact of trauma and its related disabilities. Any disability should be documented clinically and if possible with images. This description is specially important to distinguish lesions originally related to trauma from those secondary to surgical complications or clinical evolution. A detailed report can be a reference for compensation inquiries.

In summary, documentation is an important tool for:
- Diagnoses
- Interpreting clinical progress
- Assessing complications
- Assessing end results
- Epidemiological insights
- Research
- Quality control
- Medicolegal inquiries

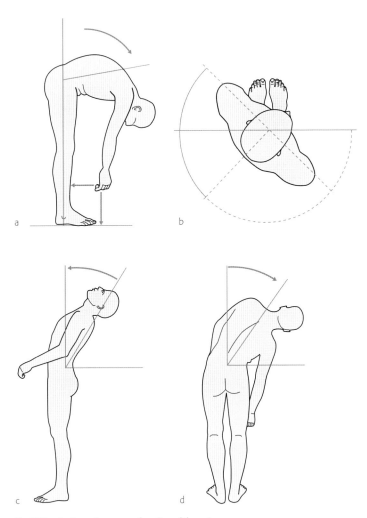

Fig 16-2a–d   Assessing range of motion of the spine.

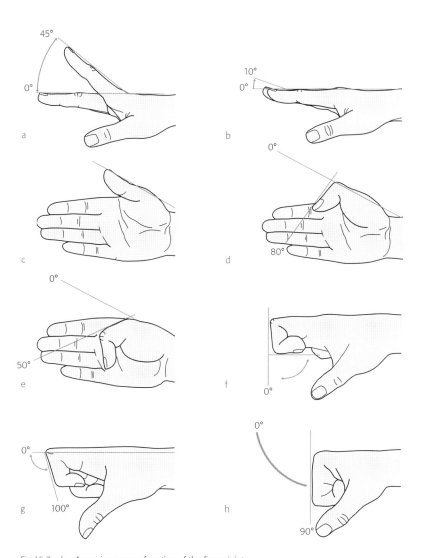

Fig 16-3a–h Assessing range of motion of the finger joints.

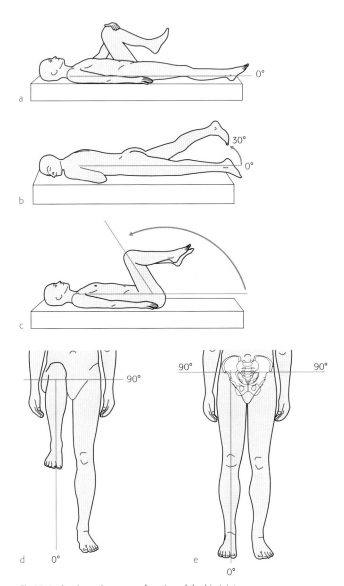

Fig 16-4a–h   Assessing range of motion of the hip joint.

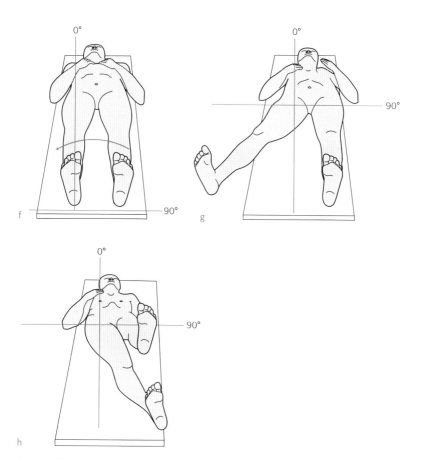

Fig 16-4a–h (cont) Assessing range of motion of the hip joint.

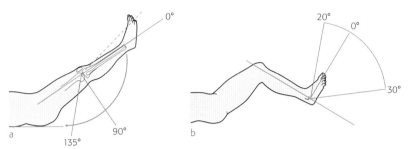

Fig 16-5a–b   Assessing range of motion of the knee and ankle joints.

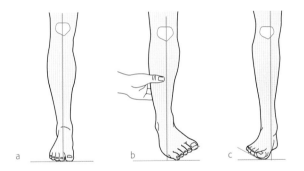

Fig 16-6a–c   Assessing range of motion of the ankle and foot
joints in inversion and eversion.

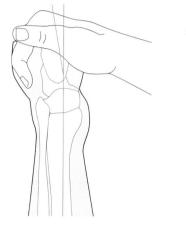

c

Fig 16-7a–c Assessing range of motion of the subtalar joint in abduction and adduction.

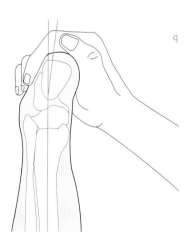

b

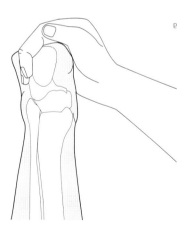

a